BECOMING
THE *BEST*
YOU

With The Hodgsons
REVISED EDITION

ELLY AND RYAN HODGSON

ELLY & RYAN HODGSON

REVISED EDITION, DECEMBER 2020

BECOMING THE *BEST* YOU:-REVISED

CONTENTS

WHO IS THIS FOR?

THIS BOOK is for you if you've struggled to achieve goals whether they be health and fitness related, career, or any life goals really, for some time now, perhaps it has felt like all your life you have been on some kind of journey to make progress, only to find 'life' or just 'stuff' has got in the way and slowed you down'. Maybe you've followed nearly every form of diet, followed what the latest trend is, only leaving you to feel fed up, frustrated, annoyed, even a little bit angry about how you've tried all these 'methods' or programs, and either have seen some short-term results or none at all, often they've always promised the world and unfortunately not delivered it.

Have you possibly struggled with your goals because of the choices you made because of not valuing your worth? Perhaps find yourself making decisions that actually take you further from your goals as opposed to toward them.

This book will show you the reasons why they've not worked in the past and also show you how to counteract them and work towards long-term, sustainable success because we know there's no point in the temporary methods that leave you the way you're feeling now.

We know your ultimate goal is to be the **best version of yourself** and to become the best version of yourself, we have created a 4 step process that has worked for THOUSANDS of our clients over the last 5 years

So whatever your goal or goals are, this book will provide you with our process to self-realisation of what you are capable of.

THANK YOU.

We know it's the 'norm' to do the thank you at the end of the book, which we will, however, we want to say a thank you to you for investing time, energy and money in yourself. You will not regret it. Read this through to the end and follow the key steps and we know it will work for you like it has for the 1000s of men and women we have helped on our programmes.

WHO ARE WE?

We are Ryan and Elly of Hodgson Health, an online coaching company that specialises in helping busy men and women become the best version of themselves, but more importantly, improving their relationship with themselves. We have been working at this for the last 5 years online and have helped over 4000 people with 'The Best YOU Formula'.

We will go through our four key principles that make up the Best YOU Formula to help you become the best version of yourself and see why you are a priority.

We feel only if you get these four things correct can you sustainably expect to be happy with yourself. Have one of these four things missing, and unfortunately, any results will be short-lived.

It is also worth noting that you need to want to change and truly value how much being happy means to you, and this is going to be the first step.

We decided to revise our original book after the amount of amazing feedback we had when it first launched. We know now, 4 years later, this will only help even more people create clarity in their life.

Our experience in the industry has shown us how often we can chase the 'shiny' objects that create instant gratification, our job is to bring things back to what;'s really important-

Being happy and Healthy.

Watching how many men and women have been misled chasing the material things that often don't last, it really made us become more aware how it was not all about physical things such as diet and exercise, or even more weight or shape but that many factors will influence us and maybe determine our decision making which is why we coach more on a holistic approach to health and happiness rather than just focusing on fitness alone.

We look at any type of progress as unsuccessful if you have to do it again, no matter how long after you achieve it. That is why we are all about making sure the results you see **last you a lifetime**.

We think our message is simple, and it is ultimately you are trying to be the best, the best version of yourself. By this, it's not just physical which of course for some being the best version for them is predominantly revolved around.

However, the mental side of things and psychological benefits to being happier and healthier because they're really important. When we think about being healthy, most of the time, we just think about being physically healthy.

But, if you start to look out at the bigger picture if you're to lose the weight and perhaps appear physically healthy, but you're being driven mad avoiding your favorite foods or even vital nutrients to help your body function at its best, it will not be sustainable but it's also not going to be any good for your own mental health.

So that's why it's all about making sure you have a holistic approach to health and a holistic approach to your goals. Don't just think of one area and get tunnel vision about which we will talk about, 'The 4B's' further on in this book. It's really important that you look at the bigger picture and that's what we aim to help you with during this book.

We are brutally honest coaches that with our clients because we know there is a difference between an excuse and a reason, and half of the time what we think are reasons, are really just excuses for not working towards our goals.

If something is getting in the way, ultimately it means you prioritise that thing over what your goal was, which is absolutely fine, as long as you're open about that. However, you need to knock the excuses on the head because people that have excuses don't achieve their goals. People that have excuses don't move forward.

So you have a thought now, about whether you will make excuses or whether you will find reasons that they are excuses, and you should ignore them to keep moving forward. The choice is yours. What way are you going to have it?

Are you going to be an excuse maker who stands still, because often when we 'standstill' or listen to our excuses we don't really stand still at all. We often slip further back.

Or, are you going to find ways to demolish the excuses and recognise when they're coming up into your head?

As we know the big difference between the two of them.

One thing we have always done when we speak with clients is make things as simple as possible, which is why we've come up with a simple formula to achieving goals in all areas of your life.

We know how complicated things can get. We know how confusing things can get for you, particularly when you just want to lose weight, we mean, how difficult should it be?

What's the right thing to do?

What's the wrong thing to do?

Everywhere you look, something that you thought was right is being said it's wrong. So many things you perhaps thought were right, you're now hearing is wrong and visa versa. We aim to make this as simple as possible. Follow the framework and you will progress. Go towards the end of this book, and you will read our daily practices. If you follow these straight off from day one, you will see progress. However, we always encourage you to read the whole book to understand a bit more about how we've come up with the best YOU formula.

We developed this formula after working with thousands of clients during our time in the industry so far. Because we wanted to find the simple, sure-fire way to help you achieve your goals without you feeling like it's all too much and takes away from other areas in your life.

Because we have a strong belief that everyone has a right to make progress and be happy and healthy.

So this is aimed to try to simplify that. It is impossible for us to put everything on paper in this short book, but we hope this will give you an insight and make it a lot simpler for you in the long run.

Now, remember these are just words on paper and you **actually have to do the work** to see the progress, reading this and doing nothing means we've failed too.

Do you believe in overnight success?

We really don't believe there is such a thing as 'overnight success'. In fact, no real success comes without hard work, grit and determination. When you see these success stories, you normally just see a start and an end point, which is fine. But, these people that got this success' have been on a journey. They've done the work; they've walked the walk.

They've faced their own challenges. They faced their own difficulties, and they've probably faced the choice or the thought of quitting many times because ultimately, success comes from hard work.

There are no shortcuts.

There is no one-way ticket.

Unfortunately, when you hit success, you need to work hard to maintain it and stay successful because there isn't such a thing as an overnight success or luck when it comes to true success.

Do the work and keep moving forward.

So we can imagine that the fact that you've bought this book tells us that this probably isn't the first time you've tried to work towards your goals

In fact, you've probably tried on many occasions to push towards these goals? Perhaps seeing this short-term success and sometimes perhaps not even the slightest bit of progress. And it definitely frustrated you for some time, so now, you need to know the best way forward.

Not only is now enough is enough of living with frustration, but the time has come to make this permanent solution, because if you don't, the battle within yourself that never goes away, the things you tell yourself, the way you walk into a room is all affected as are those around you (even if you think they aren't). We want to help change that so you can be kind with your thoughts, which you will see by the end of this book is life-changing not only for you but the ones you care about too.

But first, there's something we want you to know before you read on in this book.

Your goals are really important, and we value them.

They're so important we want you to hold them at the forefront of your mind whilst you read this book because if you don't, you've wasted your time in even reading it. We will cover goal setting with a purpose shortly too, if you don't quite know what goals you have, but just know you want to progress, we get that, and your progress is still important.

Remember that goals are set to challenge us and there will be internal resistance at times. In fact right now, accept that you are a set of habits and in order to change or adapt to who and where you are, you need to make some changes or adaptations, and that will be tough.

Because if it were easy, you wouldn't have bought this book. If it was easy, you wouldn't have tried to make progress, and failed, on several occasions and not seen the success you were happy with. In fact, if it was easy, we wouldn't have jobs, and certainly wouldn't have written this book. That's why we want you to remember your goals, how important they are, and recognise that there will be some work involved, and yes, you are worth it and you deserve it.

So carry on reading to find out more about how exactly is the best way to go about it.

Have you ever used the comment "she's so lucky" when talking about someone who's perhaps a little further along their journey than you?

We wanted to mention this because we often find that using luck as an excuse can really demoralize you and make you feel like the people who have achieved results have something you don't. Because ultimately, there is no luck involved.

There is no such thing as luck unless you look at it in the way that we do, that the harder you work, the more committed you are, the luckier you'll get.

So, bearing that in mind when you start on your journey. Luck will have very little to do with it, and we don't want to 'fluff' things up to be lucky.

Yes, you might have a little 'bad luck' if your hormones are really all over the place, which makes you struggle to lose weight, or perhaps something happens outside of your control that sidetracks you that could be 'bad luck'. But, we can do things to try to impact or reduce the impact that anything external will have on your progress towards your goals. You are the driver on your own journey.

We want to make this clear from the offset- One of the most important skills for being the best version of yourself definitely has to be patience. You need to have an element of patience for doing it in a sustainable way, that's for sure.

Because nothing worth having comes easy. We know if it were easy, everyone would do it, and we would have everyone feeling 'successful' all the time. When asked most don't feel truly successful.

You don't want a quick fix. If you wanted a quick fix you'd have bought one fad out there that you've probably tried in the past and recognized that they don't work long term.

Give yourself time and focus on little wins every day.

A Question

Are you on this cycle of success, to give up to failure to start again? We see many of this in 'our world'.

Are you working hard day in, day out to see progress and not really getting anywhere?

Static, you're going nowhere fast, and you're not feeling any better, even the bits of progress you've made slip back when 'life' takes over. Trust us when we say you're not alone. We've seen it, we've seen it time and time again. Don't stay on the 'revolving door' that is frustrating to say the least.

Throughout this book, it is really important for you to understand one thing before you even start.

We have the philosophy that if you give a boy a fish, they'll eat for a day. But, teach him to fish, he'll eat for the rest of his life. That's why shortly, we will help to know and understand how and why you're making progress too, this isn't a going through the motions kind of thing. No 'trust the process' coaching here because we've seen it time and time again.

So perhaps you're a busy mum with young kids to feed. You're working, trying to do the housework, look after the husband. Then you've got to get uniforms ready for the next day. Then you've got to try to think about how you will get your exercise in, how you will prepare your food, how you will give yourself some time to actually help you lose weight.

Or perhaps, you are a busy working man or woman, never switching off from work, it has never been a 9am - 5pm job, you don't take lunch breaks, you grab what you can when you can, perhaps coffee and a chocolate bar from the vending machine gets you through the day you finally get home and the thought of making a meal is too tiresome-

Whatever your lifestyle is, we completely get it...

It becomes even more stressful when you're stressed, that affects our decisions, affecting how we feel about ourselves. It's a vicious cycle, a vicious cycle that's extremely difficult to get out of and eventually becomes a habit.

That's life.

Just because you have a goal in mind, that doesn't mean the world will stop. It doesn't mean you can forget about the housework, the washing the clothes, the meals, the kids, the family, the to-do lists at work, perhaps staffing issues. Unfortunately, it doesn't work like that. If only it did, then making progress would be 10 times, in fact, a billion times easier. Well, life carries on, things still need to be done.

We still need to go to work, and we still need to ultimately fulfill our life role. That makes life a hell of a lot harder because we know demands are so high on an average person nowadays. This is why it's even more important to make sure we get everything put in place before we even start.

When you're in the search for progress, you can often get so drawn into — you must make that little bit of progress here and this little bit there and often lose touch with how you're actually feeling and you're pulling yourself in all sorts of different directions.

Which we find absolute madness because, ultimately, surely your main goal is to just feel better about yourself, whether that is being lighter, being in better shape, being a better parent, being more wealthy, is what would make you feel better. It doesn't really matter as long as you're feeling better. And that should always be your ultimate goal.

What's the point in loads of progress and feeling like death? Answers on the postcard.

During this book, our aim is not to help you do more to become the best version of you... **It's aimed to help you to do less, but better.** So, by this, we mean, we know that if you get a few key fundamentals correct, then that means it will make a minimal (negative) impact to your life to see more sustainable change as opposed to doing more and more that you can't sustain, we mean, you're already busy, right?

Because we've seen it before with people doing long, mundane, workouts and on super strict diets, working 12+ hours a day and we know that it doesn't work long term, never has done, never will do. So, like we said, we want you to be doing less, but more intelligently. We're sure you're already busy enough as it is, without having more to do?

Right now, there are so many ways to simplify our lives. We as a society are creating convenience, yet we want to add more burden at the same time, it's kind of backwards.

It's clear that people are becoming more and more conscious of their overall health. One aspect of being healthy will include being mentally healthy, and that can be linked closely to being happy which is sure the primary goal of goal setting?

In theory, making progress is easy, but in practice, it's a different story altogether. It's far from easy to make progress if you don't have a clear plan and clear goals.

That's why we, as coaches have a job. That's why the coaching industry is growing every single week, every single month, of every single year. Because more and more people are struggling to create clarity and move forward.

We find that most of the programs out there were extremely complex and difficult to follow from our views and experience and feedback from our clients. We are often expecting 'real-life' people to live in the gym or perhaps function on a fraction of the calories we would set. Or even worse focus so much on one area of their life that others slip back.

We see, complicated diet plans with recipes that take hours to cook, complicated workouts that involve doing exercises that the majority of people trying to lose weight can't do combined with spending hours a day trying to 'get active; when they're already busy.

We realised that more and more people need help on what to do more simply. More people need to understand that making progress in any area, in fact all areas, can be relatively simple when it's done in the right way. So throughout this book, we will go through the four key principles to the best YOU formula for long-lasting results. People don't need more information, you don't need more information. In fact, people often have too much information they don't really know what to do with it.

Just do a Google search of the quickest way to <achieve said goal> and you'll find over a million results within half a second. It's a crazy amount of information at our disposal, yet we as a society are still struggling to create clarity.. This is why we know people need one thing and **that's action.**

Without action, nothing will happen, and there are millions of ways to make progress and make it slightly different to the last thing you tried, But, the reality is any of them will probably work if done with the right format and the **mindset is right** and the lifestyle is right because these are the two most important things.

Goal setting with a purpose-

Truth is throughout our time in the coaching realm and since we wrote the first edition of this book we've come across and worked with literally thousands of people who tend to miss out on this step. We mean, there's setting goals, then there's setting goals **with a purpose.**

When setting a goal in any area of your life it's important to delve deeper into understanding why that goal is important to you. We will share with 'the 4B' in which to set goals shortly in this book. However right now, say you have a goal, we want to delve into your mind to establish why it's important.

So we ask the why 5 times, this is called the 5 whys, which many coaches will use. When we do that, we often discover the reason we actually thought we were setting the goal wasn't the reason after all.

The why is never the why.
So when you're about to set a goal, ask yourself:-

Why is that important?
Why is that important to you?
Why is that important to you?

[19]

Why is that important?
And why is that important?

This doesn't always have to be asked 5 times, it could be more, it could be less, but the key here is that you get to a reason that is truly important to you.

For us, whenever we set goals with our health and fitness, why is almost always, Aoife-Mae (6) and Niamh (2) nearly every time.

Now the reason it's important to do this 'activity' is at times as you're working toward your goals there will be internal resistance as we've already mentioned. You're going to leave your comfort zone. When you leave your comfort zone, your brain is going to try and bring you back into it. This is why when we need to have that emotional connection to our why.

When you're connected with your why, that why will be so important. Giving up will no longer be an option. Because let's face it, how many times have you started on a goal that you did really want to achieve and let things slip?

Well, we'd guess you just weren't connected with your why. So before you read much further on we want you to take time to connect with your why. It's uncomfortable at times but it will change your life:

We will always remember when Elly competed as a goal of overcoming her own barriers, she would literally be brought to tears when she connected with her why. When asked why several times we came to this-

'Because, I want Aoife-Mae to grow up with a role model to look upto who's full of confidence, not one who's letting her confidence hold her back'.

Every day for months Elly connected with that; we also have many of our clients on our total transformation +1 programme literally 80% of our weekly calls come down to connecting with their why.

So don't skip this part. Read the bit about the 4Bs then get to work on this-

The 5whys, then hold that why in your mind as you read through this book.

Let's get emotional together.

The 4Bs to prevent tunnel vision:-

The 4Bs is something we've used for quite some time really, but it's only since the start of 2020 that we put a label to it.

However, before we explain them, we use the 4Bs because when you set a goal in any area of your life, it should **add value to it, not take it away.**

In fact, that's really important. We will write it again- any time you set a goal in your life, it should add value, not take it away.

Now, when we've worked with our clients, one thing we've found is often when working towards a health and fitness goal, it often takes away from other areas of their life.

So we have them set goals in all 4 areas so that they can, **Track> Assess> Adapt** on an ongoing basis.

Doing this prevents tunnel vision that many coaches and programmes appear to almost encourage when they are like, get up early to workout and sleep less, don't drink alcohol, skip the start and dessert when eating out.

Look at January, every year many people set themselves goals with their weight or the first B- 'body'. Often hitting the gym or training really hard, being strict on their diet, so their social life suffers, their relationships suffer (Besties), even their career (Business) too as they try to focus on their body-related goal. So we want to create goals in these 4 areas and use the 3 step formula to achieve these goals too.

So the 3 steps we've already mentioned are:-

Track:- track where you are on everything relevant to your goal. Now we live in a technological world where there are apps for everything, however, a good quality journal (invest money in one) is just as effective. You want to be able to track where you are and where you're heading.

Assess:- where you are periodically, is it going in the right direction? Assess the very same things you're tracking you have data on these things now and we often say, data or stats don't lie. Women, for physical, 'Body' goals, let's do this monthly at the same point in your cycle and look at the progress made, physically and emotionally in all 4 areas.

Adapt:- note that this isn't change, it's simply adapting what you're already doing, as opposed to changing. This helps you make sure it works for you and fits your lifestyle. You also make it easier to know what adaptations have worked and what hasn't.

So now we move onto the 4Bs. Now the truth is, many people will skip this part and think-

'I don't need to set goals on this'
'I'm reading this book to help me lose weight'
'This part isn't for me'

Now, if you do that, unfortunately, you have only got yourself to blame if you don't make the progress you want. Or even worse, you make progress in one area only to find other areas have slipped. Take note of the 4Bs and make sure you set goals in each area and do the 5 whys exercise for each of them.

Before we go on to them, remember a goal could be to maintain one area of your life whilst making more progress on another, but it's still a goal nonetheless.

Body:- when it comes to the body goals, this can be your weight, your shape, your appearance, or even your fitness levels.

This generally tends to be the area that many can set goals with ease, setting them with purpose is perhaps not so easy.

So that weight loss goal or clothes size goal is the body goal, and only one of the parts of your life. We will say numerous times throughout this book, you are more than a weight on the scales, more than a clothes size and more than body shape.

Brain:- This is arguably the most important one when it comes to goals because realistically, if you achieve your brain goals you'll probably find that the rest of them fall into place **because the mind leads the body**. So let's set goals with your brain, and these are more about how you feel about yourself, how you talk about yourself, the message you give to yourself. A lot of the work we do with our clients is linking the brain and the body goals to ensure the body goal-related progress comes from a position of self-love.

Example:- 2 people with the same goal, to lose 3 stone. Person 1, hates their body, so decides to cut their calories extremely low, and beast it with excessive exercise. Person 2, on the other hand, starts to look at their body, and show it the love and respect it deserves so they nourish it with nutrient-dense foods and good activity levels. Both will lose the weight, but the emotional progress they make, how they feel at the end will be completely different. We will leave you to decide which route you want to go down here. If it's person 1, stop the world we want to get off. You've got the wrong book in your hands.

Besties:- This is your relationships, those people around you. Not just intimate relationships like your partner, but your children, family, friends, work colleagues and anyone else who is part of your life.

When we deliver our goal settings with purpose webinars to corporate clients we categorise things when it comes to setting goals and besties or relationships is one under the really important section. It often raises questions but when that internal resistance kicks in, your besties should be by your side to help. But also, long after you achieve your goals, your besties will be there.

So set goals with these, it could be setting coffee dates, finding ways to show you love someone, ensuring you have an affectionate relationship. Making sure you don't become 'one of them couples' that doesn't have sex anymore.

It could even be setting the goal of not shouting at your kids as much, we've both used this one to pretty much eliminate shouting in the TeamHodgson household.

The goal here is to make conscious efforts to improve the relationships that are important in your life. Do that? And you're winning.

This will also improve the overall quality of your life and again link closely to your brain. Often setting physical goals, like weight loss can end up a selfish thing, which is why setting these 'bestie' goals will help keep this adding value, never taking away.

Business:- this is relating to your 'professional role' and your finances.

So whether you have a high flying corporate role, are a stay at home mum, or recently lost your job, it's important to set goals in this area too.

Much of our 'daily life' is spent 'on our business', even if you don't have a specific job right now. We'll hazard a guess your finances are important.

If you have a job to pay the bills, we'd hazard a guess you need to keep that job or find one that offers more fulfillment in your life. Often people will say that their finances or their career aren't important, maybe you're one of the people? You need this goal most then. Look at it like this, most jobs say work 8 hours a day that's about half of your waking day so it must provide fulfillment for sure.

So take time to ask yourself, where are my finances and career heading? Where would I like them to head? Set goals that are relevant to you and then delve into why they're important.

If it's to get a particular professional qualification for example, why is that important to you? Ask it 5 times and discover the value it'll add to your life.

So now that we have the 4Bs, we will delve into the best YOU formula in just a minute, but before we do, take note:-

There will be times where a specific goal may take up more of your attention and focus, this is normal.

Just make sure you **regularly track, assess and adapt** to ensure that the decision to focus more on one area, doesn't totally forget the others and the decision to do that is a conscious one.

Okay? So now you've got goals to do with your **body, brain, besties and business,** and you've delved into 'the why' for each one and know it's important to you, in your journal? Right?

If not, stop reading and do this, please don't skip it. It's quite simply life-changing and life change does require work...

Done that now? Ok.

Now we get into the best you formula very soon, but before that, we wanted to cover something to do with the body goals because we regularly get asked about BMI or Body Mass Index. So it's important we put our stance on it in this book.

BMI EXPLAINED

BMI is something that is so widely used when we're talking about weight loss and body mass index, in short, is basically where you categorize someone as, underweight, healthy, overweight, obese or morbidly obese, based on just their height and weight.

So if they're heavier than what people might perceive as healthy, they're overweight, and people can take this as gospel, so one could go to a doctor, be in good health, however have slightly more more muscle and be deemed overweight and be told they need to go on a calorie deficit in order to be 'healthy'.

However, the health and fitness industry and even now the health industry more specifically are moving further and further away from using body mass index as a safe guide to being a 'healthy weight' because people are all different shapes and sizes and ultimately people who have a wider frame will probably weigh slightly more than somebody who has got a narrower frame even if they're the same height.

It doesn't mean one of them is healthier than the other. That's why we want you to really remove that focus from the weight as such and focus more on how you feel, because if you have weight to lose, and you follow all the guidelines in this book, the weight will come off, that we are sure of.

Weight loss is a by-product of becoming the best version of you if that's what your body needs.

But, if it's more shape change you want, you'll change shape but may not necessarily lose weight. That's something we want you to remember, that ultimately, your body will respond in the right way provided you follow the correct mindset, lifestyle, nutrition and exercise.

So keep that in the front of your mind as you read on and we hope that you will enjoy reading this book and take some serious notes away from it.

You will learn the simplest way that, we know, works to lose weight, and keep it off, and we believe the most important one is the mindset.

After mindset comes close second is a lifestyle.

Then we will go onto nutrition, and then finally activity, which in the first edition of this book we called exercise which we will explain why we have adapted this word as we get on to that section of the book..

We know most people almost always do this in reverse when starting their health goals and focusing on diet and exercise.

We feel strongly that the fitness industry, at the moment, is failing as a whole and ultimately failing you. It's failing people that are trying with their best intentions to lose weight and /or be healthy. With the fitness industry being just 40 years old,

People are fatter than they've ever been before.

People are getting type two diabetes more than ever before.

People are dying of heart-related and health-related issues due to being overweight more than ever before.

More people are being diagnosed with mental health issues

Women are under more pressure to look a certain way

This tells us being happy and healthy really is not as simple as just diet and exercise.

Life has changed over the last 40 years. The demands on the average person are much higher now than it's ever been. People are busier and have less spare time to dedicate to spending hours in the gym.

When trying to be healthy, there is no right or wrong way, there is just an easier way and a harder way. But what's important is the way you think and the actions you take.

IF you can take control of your mindset to understand the way you think will impact the results you will get, you will find the easier way. Fail on this step, you may see physical changes but the mind will still be back where you started and we said before, the mind leads the body, so the mind will lead you back to where you started.

That is why we feel it is really important for us to go through our 4 key principles to help you become the best version of yourself **with longevity in mind**. Before we get to the diet and exercise there are a couple of things we need to work on to see how to improve the relationship with yourself.

For us, there is no point in feeling better about yourself for a short period only to slip in confidence again just like there's no point losing weight only to put it back on. The things both need to be sustainable because out of the thousands of women we have helped over our time in the industry, we've found no one wants to lose weight only to put it back on, no one wants to get healthy to then slip backward. Maybe you are the exception? If you are. Again, you're reading the wrong book.

That's why we need to make sure that all the results we get are sustainable and achievable within their lifestyle. We hope you enjoy this book.

The Car analogy

To make an analogy to show you how important we find all four of these key principles are, we can use a car. If we look at mindset, they're the keys to the car.

You're getting nowhere without them. And then when we look at lifestyle, they're the wheels. We need the wheels to move. Then when you've got the nutrition, that's the fuel, the petrol, that's what will keep you going. Then when you go with the activity, that will be the oil to just fine-tune it and make that final touch a bit better.

One way we like to look at it when we talk to people before they work on their health and fitness goals is to remind them; the harder you have to work physically to almost force a change with your health and happiness in your life, the harder it will be to sustain it.

That's why we are so big on making sure you are doing things intelligently and having the knowledge so that it is sustainable and you haven't focused so hard on one specific area of your life that the others fall apart. Like we have seen many health and fitness professionals, bless them, focus so hard on their bodies, and look great, but unable to maintain a stable relationship and their career doesn't look too good either. We aren't here to judge though we've just seen it first hand. In fact Ryan focused so hard on his career a few years back his mental health declined and ended up suffering with depression and anxiety. It wasn't good at all. His body also suffered physically but his business was doing well, see what we mean?

But back to you, how many times have you started it? We've asked this question already, so you know the answer.

Before we became parents, I think it was safe to say, we were pretty ignorant of how much 'family life' can get in the way of yourself and blinding you to your worth.

When your primary goal is helping or providing for the family and other people around you, think about how easy it can become to lose focus on your own personal goals in any area really, like we can just kind of 'drift' dare we say?

Before Aoife-Mae was born, we really just focused on diet and exercise and everything else could fall around it, but throw a family in the mix.

Having kids or even just being in a serious relationship, other things start to take priority. That routine with your training and your nutrition that's been the focus when it comes to your goals and the lifestyle building around it easily falls to the side.

In fact, we've lost count of the number of people we've seen that got in a relationship and unfortunately put on weight, or lost the shape they were happy with which there's nothing wrong with unless it affects your confidence, your moods, and ultimately how you feel about yourself as a whole. Then eventually the relationship itself can also begin to suffer. You should feel even better about yourself when something like a new relationship happens. Remember adding value to our life, not taking it away?.

So it's important to remember this is why we always focus on mindset and lifestyle first because once you have the lifestyle and the mindset in the right place, the nutrition and activity will fall into place from there. Like think about lifestyle, that will encourage activity and the right nutrition. Right? Let's hope so by the end of this book anyway. Do it the opposite way, though, you're setting yourself up for a long battle with yourself and just 'life' — a battle ultimately that's ten times harder to win than if you get it right the first time around.

SIDENOTE:- When embarking on a health and fitness journey, the worst thing you can do is to compare yourself to other people. Even if you've got a friend who's got a similar starting point and you're doing the same thing.

Because ultimately, it can really and probably will, deflate one of you. Yes, sometimes it will help you, competition and comparison may work positively. However, we find 80% of the time comparing yourself to other people because you will end one way, and it will not be with a smile. We often only hear about 'success stories' so if you're sitting there comparing your worst moments or downfalls to another person's successes that's not going to help you in any way, shape or form.

We want you to focus more on yourself and that's why mindset is so important because **it's all about you and having your mind in the right place** to help you move forward. Forget anyone else and focus solely on you.

Before we move on, there's one thing we'd like to make clear from the offset is regardless of how much progress you'd like to see in any area of your life, we need to improve the relationship with yourself and understand why you feel the way you do.

THE REAL REASON

Ultimately your goal is as important to you as you make it.

So by this we mean it doesn't matter what your goal is unless you prioritise it. Yes, it will probably see more profound health benefits if you're someone who's got five stone to lose versus someone who has 5lbs to lose. That will help as a motivating factor.

But, ultimately it's all about our priorities and how we prioritise things in our lives. So that's why we want to make sure you sit down, **assess your life**, and ultimately assess the importance of our goals to you.

And it boils down to us and how we prioritise working towards that goal.

Before we go any futher, we want to make this very clear, from the very offset.

You do not need anyone else's permission to try to become the best version of yourself.

We'd encourage writing this down DAILY.

"I do not need anyone else's permission to be the best version of myself'
That's right you really do not need anyone else's approval or validation in your pursuit of trying to become the best version of yourself. We feel it's vital you remind yourself of this every second of every day, and the reasons behind exactly why we feel it's important will become clear further into this book.

Now, the reason we want to highlight this is because we find, a vast majority of the people we work with when looking for personal development of any kind, be it with their body, brain, business or besties will ask or look for permission from others, to better themselves.

To try and become that best possible version. We've lost track of the number of women who want to lose weight, talk to us and need to just 'run it by their husband', and unfortunately he doesn't see the value in it.

So if you're somebody that needs permission, you've got children and you feel guilty for wanting to lose weight, or get healthier, and dedicate a bit of time to you, don't.

[34]

You deserve this, and not only that, *when you invest in yourself, everyone else will benefit around you too.* And if people around you can't see the benefit of it, perhaps the issue is theirs, not yours. So, let's read on, and really make some serious progress guilt-free. No one should feel guilty for wanting to be the best version of themselves.

We'll probably say that at various points throughout this book. It might sound like a broken record, but we cannot underestimate how important this is.

Something we think people often do wrong is work on physical related goals for a time, for specific dates. And by this, we mean we have literally lost count of the number of people who see us because they want to lose weight for their wedding day, or they want to lose weight for their holiday.

And we completely get it; it's always good to have a deadline for your goal.

But, let's forget about losing weight for a set day and let's look at why you are struggling with confidence right now?

Let's look at the mindset that is telling you it will all change when you are a set amount of weight lighter on the scales. Let's look at that mindset that seems to tell you you're worth more as a human being when you are in a smaller bikini; seems mad when we write it like that, right? Then we start to see that, the weight is less important, the dress size is less important, and in fact if we do change shape or lose weight, we do it for life. Because all 'life progress' should always be permanent.

If you are trying to make progress on a specific date and you don't care if you then slip back, this book really isn't for you. We only want to help people that are going to progress in a sustainable way that fits your lifestyle and again **adds value**. We can't stress enough the importance of doing that.

Not only will you feel better about yourself for a longer-term but the health and happiness benefits are much better.

STARTING OFF ON THE RIGHT FOOT

FOR US AND OUR clients, when we're working with them, we make it clear that their goal is not a destination. It's not something that you hit and stay there, work needs to continue to be done otherwise you move away from it. You must have heard that saying *'success is never owned, it is rented, and rent is due every day'* well it's true we are afraid to say.

It's ultimately a journey.

Self-progress of any type is a journey because everything we do fits our lifestyle, and your lifestyle is a journey. It's not something that has an end.

It's not something that has an expiry date, and it's important to understand that from the start because when you achieve that goal if you take your foot off the gas, what happens next?

Answers are on a postcard.

That's why we want you to really, really think about your journey rather than your destination, so aim to enjoy it. That way even if you don't get to your goal or 'destination', if you're on a good journey that you enjoy, you're going to have made progress and be a lot closer to the end of it.

Keep moving forward. Stay on track, follow the steps in this book to commit to yourself that you're going to get towards your goals in a safe, and sustainable manner.

That ultimately is what this whole book is about. If you don't want to face a sustainable journey, don't read this book because you're wasting your time. Pass this to someone else who wants sustainable life progress

Example:-How many times have you tried to lose weight or started to lose weight, put it all back on and then go and set yourself the same goal again? Because when you give up or throw the towel in on a particular program, it doesn't mean you will settle and suddenly become happy with where you are now, regardless of how that programme made you feel.

You will never be happy with that. That goal you had will still be there in the back of your mind, eating away at you. That's why we have the saying, **do it right or do it twice.** This thought process is simple and kind of obvious, right? We mean to lose weight the right way, i.e., it doesn't go back on, or you never have to do it twice. If you have to lose weight twice, you did it wrong. Same with your relationships, career and mindset too, you don't want to make progress to let it slip back over and over again, right?

It doesn't get any easier the more and more you start, stop, start again, unfortunately, practice doesn't make perfect either. The more and more times you give up or falter, you make giving up become easier and easier.

When people talk about self-progress, more often than not, it's ruled by physical things for example, many of our clients on weight loss journeys they will base their whole success and how they feel about their day, week or month etc on the weight they weigh when they step on the scales, which is something we want to come far, far away from, has your day ever been determined by something as simple as what the scales say? Well, we want you to know you're more than scales or anything physical. Happiness needs to be coming from within.

We want you to ask yourself this question before you read on in any part of this book, and that is, are you being truthful to yourself?

Are you being honest about what your goals really are and **why they're important to you?**

The reason we want you to ask this question is most people don't bother answering it correctly. Most people will say their goals are important to them.

However, the life they lead, the reality is it would suggest very different. That's why we want you to sit back, answer that question before you read on, and only when you've answered that question should you continue to read this book and make your self progress.

Weight Loss vs Fat loss

When working with our clients, we feel it is really important to show the difference between weight loss and fat loss because ultimately, what most people want is fat loss. If you're to look at most women, they'll fluctuate in weight over the course of their 28-day cycle (variable depending on your cycle), sometimes up to 9 or 10 pounds, for example. This doesn't mean they've put on 9 or 10 pounds and lost it in a month. It means they retain slightly more water due to their hormones. Yet this can still affect how women feel about themselves. Also, women can seriously suffer from lower self-esteem in the later parts of their cycle.

This is why we tend to focus more on how you feel as opposed to a weight on the scales on any given day. With body goals, yes, it's great to have physical goals, but we would always encourage making them more about shape, perhaps body fat percentage over a specific weight. Shape change and how you actually feel rather than weight loss being the main focus. It's important to mention that muscle takes up much less room than fat. Fat is much less dense, which means it will weigh less if you have the same volume of muscle as fat. Muscle is firmer too. We have yet to find somebody that says fat looks more attractive than muscle, surely you'd agree?

In modern society, we put so much pressure on ourselves to have a certain appearance. You only have to look around on various forms of social media to see it. You look around on the internet at so many ways to enhance the way we look. Whether it is through filters when we put photos up to waist trimmers that make us look thinner to extreme fad diets and ridiculous amounts of exercise. All of these in pursuit of looking better or 'good' using that term loosely, with very little regard to actually being healthy or feeling healthy. And that's the most important thing for us all, surely. It is to be healthy and happy of course.

Now more often than not when we do these things we are being unhealthy. Even when you look at things such as filters, they are giving us all an unhealthy perception of what people 'should' look like.

They put pressure on people to look a certain way when it's not true.

It's not reality.....

The reality is, we are all different shapes and sizes and it's about us all accepting that. Yes, we can put work in improving the way we look. But, that should not come at the costs of feeling worse or feeling false and giving out a false message.

It sends the wrong message out to those around us our children and younger generations, when ultimately, the only thing we are really doing is pushing ourselves further and further away from health and happiness. Yes it may give us the instant gratification of a few more likes, but when we sit and think about it- getting likes for this false message, surely that's worse than no likes at all?

You are fooling yourself and only building up more insecurity when you feel like you need to use these filters to get a certain appearance, when you feel like you need to use these waist trimmers to have a certain appearance. When you feel like you need to use these fad diets to get into a certain appearance.

It's all false.

The other choice, you can either be truthful to yourself, yes, it may be uncomfortable at first, but it's much easier to stick to, and much more fulfilling that we are sure of. Then do things in life and focus on being healthy and let the shape change and/or weight loss look after itself safely or keep lying to yourself and live an unhappy life with your appearance or shape. The choice is yours.

For health and fitness in general, it's really important to understand that there is absolutely no one size fits all and we shouldn't measure our size with someone else's ruler.

So by this we mean, you are unique. You have your own unique goals, your own unique reasons and your own unique lifestyle. Then add your own unique mindset. This is why everything should be catered towards you and specifically towards you.

Throughout this book, we are going into more depth about exactly how we can do that to make sure that things are specific to you, even if you are doing it with somebody else.

So what if we said to you, do this program and you will lose weight? But you will be tired, irritable, suffer from headaches, and feel sick all the time.....

Because the reality is, these are the side effects that we regularly seen being described by people who have tried some of these quick fixes out there where they replace their meals with shakes and one size fits all programmes.

Yes, these people are losing weight, but ultimately, they feel worse than they did when they started. The only slightly positive thing is that they weigh less on the scales, even if they don't look any better physically. They look grey, run-down, and ultimately look a little malnourished. They've taken their relationships for granted, taken their own happiness for granted and their own natural defences to detoxify and defend any illness, not to mention their mental state- you get the picture, right? Perhaps you're nodding right now? Most people have a weight or shape goal to FEEL BETTER. Why do they take an option that makes them feel worse?

We are urging you to look at any time, money and energy you spend on your health and wellbeing as investing in yourself properly so you do something that will **last a lifetime with you.**

You will not be doing these quick fixes and finding yourself a year from now setting yourself the same goals you've set when you first started this because that's exactly what's happening, we see it daily, and it really upsets us as coaches that focus on **Health and Happiness.**

It's a vicious cycle. That's why many quick-fix methods still have a business because they know you'll lose weight with them. The weight will go back on, you'll think to yourself, how did I lose that weight the last time? And head straight back for that quick fix.

We need to be wiser about this. We need to understand a little more about the real effects it will have on your body. Your metabolic rate, your output, your hormones your fertility will be affected because you opted for a quick fix. That's not mentioned in any extreme plan. That's not in the guidelines. That's not in the benefits of these quick fixes. It's not in the before and after photos of someone who's made HUGE changes in a short amount of time.

Throughout various points in this book, you'll see us emphasise the importance of understanding and how understanding is one of the fundamentals of any form of self-progress.

It's like if you ever watch children when told to do something, they often are reluctant to do it, however, when it's explained why and they understand it, their whole attitude will change. It's the same for us as adults too.

You need to understand everything from why you are where you are right now in life, why you're in the current shape, you're in now to why you want to be a better version of yourself, what that means to you, and how to get there.

We know only when you actually understand it and have the knowledge can it be sustainable. That's why we're such huge believers in having an understanding rather than just going through a program to see progress. We know some coaches/mentors use this phrase 'trust the process, fu5k that! We want to understand the process too.

That's why we're so big on people taking a bit longer to learn and understand it. We don't want you to just go through a plug and play program that one size fits all because **you're unique.**

So follow the advice we give you in this book and this WILL just help to make sure you get the best results. That not only will be there for the short-term but for the long-term too. So you don't need to read this book again in a few years' time when the progress you've made across the 4Bs has slipped back.

When starting out on your Self progress journey (yes we're calling it that now), as we've mentioned it's really important to track and assess progress in more than just one way. So by this, we mean to break down the goals in the 4Bs, and track progress with each one in more ways than one. With the Body it could be weight, shape, energy, with the Besties it could be sex life, closeness or even not arguing, with them don't just focus on one thing as it can be misleading and affect your overall level of happiness and after all that's the aim of the game right?

Lastly, write somewhere, that is private to you how you feel about yourself even out of 10 how happy you are, 0 being the lowest and 10 being the highest and then again each month review your thoughts, this will help you to level things out, particularly with women you can feel very different at different points in your cycle, So try to do this at the same point. Like Elly struggles with self-esteem in the later stages of her cycle, when her testosterone levels have dropped and her period is about to start, assessing then vs. day 10-12 would be rather pointless and not a true representation of progress.

So we have the tracking and assessing, we want to do things from the right perspective too particularly when we are adapting. We want you to be doing things from a place of self-respect and self-love (this may be tough right now if you've spent years hating yourself). We want you to realise that the more you love something, the more you take care of it.

Think of it like this for a second.

Your children, you love them more than anything. There's nothing you wouldn't do to help them because you really love them.

We noticed that there's a direct correlation in the results people get based on how much they love themselves. And we're not just talking about loving the person or the body you're aiming to get towards because that's great.

However, **you need to love the body, mind and soul you have now,** and that can sometimes seem like a daunting feeling. That's why you really need to work on your own mindset and get your head in the right place so you can begin to love the body you have right now.

We know it is difficult, in fact since we started coaching most of the men and women we have worked with, this has been a relatively foreign concept. It will not be something that will come naturally. However, spending the time to get your mind right will really help you love yourself, and then you'll care more about it and focus more on helping you achieve those goals. PLUS then everyone around you will benefit too (write that bit down).

It simply has to start with loving yourself and loving the body and life you've got now, not six months down the line, the body you have now. And we will go on a journey with that when we go on to mindset.

LET US ASK YOU A COUPLE OF QUESTIONS

So now we will ask you a couple of questions, and we want you to write down the answers before you read on in this book:

1. What are your goals in each of the 4Bs? (with a deadline) we do this to establish your goals now is a good way to read the book and help you to use your mind to stay focused on the end goal.

2. Then, we want you to go on to ask yourself **why are these goals important to you?** This will be the foundation

for us moving onto the first 'real' chapter, which is all about mindset.

What do you REALLY want? Now, that's a serious question we need you to consider. We want you to think very deeply about the answer because very few can actually answer it deep down and know exactly what they want because they don't really give it much thought.

They don't think about the deep, underlying things they really, truly want. That's something we want you to think about before you read on. We want you to establish exactly what you want, where you want to be, and how you want to get it.

Because you need to do that before you can do anything else and move forwards toward your goal. How can you have what you want if you don't even know what you want?

Like it's understanding, what comes with what you say you want. Example, we speak to many people who want career success, however when you get them to look at the bigger picture, the time it will take for them to do the professional exams that will take them from their family or perhaps their social circles a little? Do they realise they perhaps didn't REALLY want it? With us? Good.

Ok, so we will say something now that will probably sound kind of obvious, but you also need to want the results for you. You need to want the progress for you.

The reason we point this out is that we know more often than not people are trying to achieve their results or gain progress because of other people, because of their husbands, because of their kids, because of their parents, because of their friends or perhaps they feel like they 'should' do it.

But it's rarely because they really want to progress for themselves, and that's why it's rare that results are achieved long term.

That's something we want you to think about and consider. Because if you don't want the results yourself, they will not be longer-term.

You will never be ruthlessly committed to them. Ultimately, that's exactly what we will need at times: ruthless commitment. Being committed alone isn't enough. Be ruthlessly committed, putting your goals to the forefront of everything you do. Get the point?

Now it's not saying disregard everything else but its meaning keeping your goals in mind all the time even when you may usually slip up, like the weekend, social occasions, when the alarm goes off early and you want to stay in bed an extra 20 minutes.

So we want you to really know why you want to achieve those goals. Let's use weight, for example, many people say, when they want to lose weight, it's because they're overweight. But there's got to be an underlying reason. Why does it matter if you're overweight? Why is it important to you? Because that's what will keep you going when the going gets a bit tough and the body's internal resistance to change kicks in.

It's a unique story that's yours and something that should be held onto throughout your Self progress journey. Because when the going gets tough, and it will get tough, that's what will keep you going. That's what will be the driving force behind you that keeps you committed to yourself because ultimately only you can keep yourself committed (we can help with accountability, knowledge and support but the commitment is from you).

How important are your goals? We will ask people this time and time again because nine times out of ten, the first response we're given is just 'very important'.

Then what we want to do after we've said they're very important is establish why because it's only once we look at the why can we start to recognise how important our goals really are to us.

Because, to us, if something is very important to you, you would do almost anything for it. However, people's reality and practice reflect a very different story and provide us with very little evidence to suggest that their goal is really very important.

For example, if somebody wants to lose weight, they know to lose weight, they should adapt their lifestyle to become a little more active. They should exercise regularly and eat a balanced diet. If it's very important, then that would be extremely simple to follow.

However, they'll still go out and eat rubbish foods and lead a sedentary lifestyle, say they're too busy to prep food or train, yet have time to watch the soaps on TV say they don't want to track their food in case they 'become obsessed'.

So that tells us that their goal isn't as important to them as they first suggested. Their goal isn't very important to them if they know what happens on the soaps is more important than their goal. Surely you'd agree? The soaps aren't very important in the scheme of things, right? Yet the things you say you don't have time to do are less important than them if you have time to watch them. See what we did there?

It's just something they would like to do, and there is a big difference between "I would like to do something" to "I am going to do it" and "I really want it because it's important to me", and that's why we need to dig deep.

You need to look below the surfaces, and it is uncomfortable. It will make you feel a little emotional because your goals of self-progress should be that important to you.

Now that being said, we can adapt the deadline based on what we can commit to. For example, if you want to work on your relationships but right now have a lot on with work, so can't commit too much time you may need to set the deadline back a little. Same with weight loss if you can't perhaps be as active as you'd like or have a lot on socially that may slow your progress down.

When we ask someone why they want to achieve their goal, and they tell us it's just because they want to, that tells us it's probably not really that important to them.

But if someone tells us they want to achieve their goals because they feel like absolute crap. They avoid photos with their children. They're embarrassed to be the mum at school that hides from other mums, which tells us it's really important.

That tells us they are emotionally connected to their goals. There's very little that will get in the way of them with this in mind. When they start to struggle, we will remind them of that level of importance and how they felt at the start because once they recognise that they're making progress away from the feeling like crap, the hiding, the dodging looking in the mirror.

That will keep them going. That's because it's important to them. So that's what we want you to remember when you read this book is how important are your goals to you? **In any area! Body Brain Besties Business.**

If they're not that important, that's absolutely fine, but don't lie to yourself and don't lie to those around you by saying something is really important to you, but you prioritise things that are less important.

Before you read on in this, we want you to understand that it's not an easy ride. It takes time, and it often comes from deeper underlying issues which we will help you to remain on track as you make progress.

Remember, at times you'll feel like giving up and going back to the old ways. However, this is often how you've got to where you are now. So we ask for a bit of patience and commitment to yourself to make sure you can follow through and see long-term, sustainable results.

We don't want you to come at this from a short term plan to make progress because we know it will not work. As we've asked you already, how many times have you tried to do a short-term plan in the past? Like you see online 21 days plan for all things business, body brain and besties as a quick fix approaches even like, 12 weeks, 6 months even. It needs to be long-term.

We want you to look at this as a lifestyle and adapt everything as a lifestyle as in, 'I'm doing this now because I'm going to do it forever.

If you can't do something forever, don't start it now, because it will never last. And ultimately, that means the results you will achieve will not last, and we don't want that.

Your goal is permanent, so the results need to be permanent, and that's something you need to consider before you do anything when it comes to self-progress

MINDSET

FOR US, mindset is something we had always overlooked and probably struggled with ourselves (without knowing) until we moved into the online world and started coaching with our first online coach A.J. Mihrzad (yes we have coaches too)

Mindset is the most misunderstood concept we will cover in this book, yet the most important thing we will cover. Often people think the mindset is simply just motivation or thinking positively, but there's a lot more to it.

In fact, it's only 4 years or so that we have really started to appreciate the full value of what mindset really is.

We feel it's the most important principle in order for you to make true personal progress in any area of your life. You will need to progress internally (mindset) in order to properly move forward and stay there.

If you can't get the mindset right, it will never last. But be sure from here, it's not just thinking positively, never has been and never will be. You can think positively but not have the right mindset to achieve your goals. Having the right mindset to achieve your goals means that your mind is aligned with achieving them, and your mind is focused on them and you've got your head in the right place to do so.

When you've got your head in the right place, that will cover anything else, including lifestyle, nutrition, and activity, which we'll go into further on in this book.

So really, get the mindset right, you could probably say you've got nothing else to worry about, you will achieve those goals. Not sure if you've ever heard of the law of attraction? We were introduced to this by following Bob

Proctor and it's a genuine life-changer, basically how we get what we focus on in life.

In life there will always be obstacles, there will always be negatives, and the law of attraction has shown that when we focus on them, they will only prevail. They will only come more to light. So that's why we want to harness our mind to focus on what we truly wish to, then continue to focus on it and then we will attract it.

We always question ourselves and what we can do, we had limiting beliefs and they were preventing us from achieving our goals, sometimes from even taking that first step toward them goals.

That's why it's important to understand a little about the importance of removing those limiting beliefs. Often we don't fully realise how we have limiting beliefs, but right now, that goal that you have? Solid relationship? Weight loss? Career progress? Do you truly believe you can achieve them all within your life? Often when we have these conversations with clients in TeamHodgson it's difficult to imagine, so these limiting beliefs can knock any goal before we even get to work. Oh! and by the way, it's something we can pretend to believe we have to truly believe we can achieve it. Like often when we take time to look at why a person hasn't achieved things we often find somewhere within the stumbling block is self belief or lack of, that are stopping them. So you can see this is inside the mind, mental blocks that will often prevent us from truly reaching our full potential and becoming the best version of ourselves.

As soon as we start to unlock that and work closely with clients on their mindset, we start to see the results they can achieve, improve pretty much overnight. The physical result was almost unimportant compared to the psychological results we attained. That's why we really want to stress the high level of importance of getting the mindset right from the very start.

When starting and trying to get in the right mindset, we think it's absolutely vital you remove all distractions. That's why we will ask that you literally clear everything out of your mind (the washing can wait) and spend that five minutes focusing on your goals and what we need to do to achieve them.

If there's a distraction, and you're not fully focused, you will not get in that moment and live at the moment that will help in gaining that emotional attachment to your goals.

So, remove all distractions, no TVs, no phones, no computers, no iPads or anything like that. We want you to go into a room, sit there with just a notepad and pen, that's all you need.

Before we move on, it's important we know that when working towards your goals when you're looking at your mindset, we cannot create change until you can believe that change can actually happen. Remember this point as it's really important when starting out on your goals. You simply have to believe you can achieve them first. You must believe you can.

By this, we mean you need to have the belief that you will be able to better yourself, and we have this strong thought that everybody has a responsibility to themselves to try to be the best version of themselves.

In doing so, we need to have that belief that we can better ourselves, whether that be by bettering ourselves by looking at one of the other areas in this book or even just in your general life.

We need to make sure we have that self-belief. Without self-belief, everything else fades away. There is no progress. There is no success.

Our thought process is that when setting yourself a goal, you need to **remember the reason you want to achieve that**. And no matter who you are, the reason you want to achieve that goal will probably be associated with wanting to feel better.

It might be to feel better physically; it might be to feel better mentally, emotionally. However, it's the same principle, to feel better. So, we see no point whatsoever in you trying to set yourself a goal that's going to physically, emotionally, and mentally ruin you. Sounds really obvious when we put it like that, right?

So, try to make everything you do sustainable, fun, and safe (may sound boring but crucial) from the start. Don't do something that will not be safe. We have to make sure that anything, although it sounds boring, you do, lasts for you. There's no point in trying to do something you know won't work for a longer term.

It's important to always remember that the mind and body work hand in hand. We cannot do one without the other working with it. So please don't focus all on the body which 90% of people trying to achieve their goals do.

Make sure you spend special care and attention on getting the mind in the right place before you even start anything physical because only when you have that mind in the right place is the body ever going to get what it needs.

You can try and do it the opposite way round, but we can assure you, the mind is a lot more resistant to change than the body. That's why it's even more crucial that we get that right first. Take your time, be patient, and follow the daily things we set out below (daily rituals). You will achieve your goals with time. We see many people in the weight loss world, where they chase the physical progress and see it short term, but internally they still think and act like the fat person that started the journey. No wonder the weight piles back on before long.

So the reason we'd want you to do these daily rituals is to look at it from this angle. We want you to start the day in control, not just one day, but every single day.

Now we have to admit when we started doing this Ryan was quick to say it won't work and slam or knock it before he tried, but after a few days of practicing it (properly), the improvement in focus was incredible. He thought it was a waste of time, but doing them soon made even more time in his day because of the focus.

We see this a lot with clients who are new to daily rituals, we hear all the excuses come up - 'I don't have time', 'i'm too busy', 'it won't work for me', 'writing something out? I'd rather be doing', we've heard them all and they will all be met with, results speak louder than opinions. Commit to doing this properly for 28 days and we promise you this will transform your mornings and even your life. You'll make more progress daily than you have been in weeks.

So let's start the day in control of your mindset, in control of your thought process, and ultimately, in control of your day-to-day lifestyle. Now only when you do these daily rituals can you start the day already in real control. Like how often do you wake up, and just 'crack on' with your day without thinking about what you want to achieve today?

We have seen a significant difference between people who achieve their goals and those who do not. They control what they do daily, control their lifestyle, or control their mindset.

You need to have control of all of these and by doing these daily rituals, it will help you get in the right frame of mind to bring your goals to the forefront of it, **every single day.** Note, this is everyday not just the days you feel like it. We often get people in a routine and they feel in control so let that slip and before they know it, they have given up control to external factors and it's tough to reign it back in.

We do this and ensure it becomes habitual. Then being in control becomes habitual too. Because we see time and time again people trying to get through their day and then gain control however, if you start the day in control, it makes it a lot easier for you from the offset.

More often than not, for the women we work with when they're trying to lose weight (which they often think is their goal at first), it's easy to get hung up on things we can't do, that we can't find time to work out or we can't find time to prepare our foods, etc rather than focusing on the things we can do.

So, for example, yes, okay we can't work out five times a week. But perhaps you can work out one day a week. Perhaps you can start to do a little more exercise, could we take the stairs rather than the lift? Maybe we could walk the school run? Maybe we could do 100 squats in the break of the TV programmes you like.

Perhaps you could start to reduce the calories a little. It's just simple little things about focusing and shifting your mindset onto focusing on things you can do, rather than dreading things you can't do.

Because we see so many times that people give up because they've become so hung up on the things they can't do, we need to focus on what you can do.

As soon as you think about can, can and can, you automatically start to create a more positive environment to help you move forward towards your goals.

DAILY RITUALS

SO WHAT DO we do for daily rituals, you may ask?

Well, it's pretty simple, firstly invest in a good quality notepad and pen (not a cheap one, you won't value it), in fact, we suggest getting that before we go into exactly what these rituals are further on in this chapter.

When we start to dig a little deeper into your mindset and thoughts and where they come from. You're probably not going to like what we've got to say. But we want you to have a little step out and think about the reasons you might not like it.

We want you to read it, so we'll put it down on this book twice.

You are a direct result of the lifestyle you've led.

As we said, we will repeat it....

You are a direct result of the lifestyle you've led.

So by this, we mean you cannot blame external factors for your current situation now. The results you have had up to now are a reflection of the mindset and lifestyle you have lived up to now. Not happy with the results? Let's address the mindset of lifestyle then. We are all in control of our own little bubble, so to speak and only when we accept that can we move forward.

Now, that doesn't mean that other factors couldn't have impacted on where you are right now. However, choices you've made, things you've done, have got you in the position you're in right now, like it or not.

Once we start to accept that and understand it, you can look into a little more depth about how we can begin to make sustainable changes.

After you've accepted that you are in the current position you are in right now because of your mindset and actions, and only your mind and actions, we can then start to look at what you will do to change it and you will sense a new sense of responsibility to yourself.

Now we've established that you will surely agree that you are responsible for moving forward with these goals.

Now that's where we now need to start to train our brains to think differently. Because ultimately, the way your brain has been thinking over the last however many weeks, months, or even years, it is what got you here, reading this book to become the best you. So we can assume you don't quite feel the best you yet.

Therefore, if we want to feel better about ourselves and become the best us we need to train our brain to think like somebody who is already where we want to be, whether that be with our business, body, brain or besties. We need to think like the goal is achieved already. It's like a visualisation that will increase your emotional connection to your goals.

This can be tough particularly if like for many, this is a new concept for you, however, bear with us, it's worth working on it and persevering. . We often say putting yourself in the position of when you've achieved that goal first like when you do the daily rituals. You learn to love yourself, because the way to get the life, body or mind you love is to love the one you already have enough to deliver it.

Now let's go over a little more depth of how we can train our brains just like any other muscle group.

You can then train your brain to think differently. As we've said, it's not an overnight thing. This is something that can take months, sometimes years, to do until it becomes natural.

Once you change these thoughts, you will think more positively about yourself, naturally, even if it's for a short period of time. This will then help you to move forwards day in, day out, which then solidifies your sense of achievement.. That's why we have our daily rituals.

Often when we discuss mindset for the first time with clients, the first thing that pops into their mind is it will be all about motivation and a bit 'happy-clappy'.

However, this is not the case but we must admit that until August 2014, we thought the exact same thing. We thought mindset was all about just making negatives positives and pretending that everything is ok all the time. But this really is not the case.

Mindset is all about fine-tuning and training the brain to think in a certain way that ultimately delivers the results you want. Remember not just physical results but the emotional ones too. Once we can do that and do it CONSISTENTLY, we can train the brain to think about our goals and think about being in that moment when we achieve our goals. Once we do that, the emotional connection to these goals will increase ten-fold.

We often say, when we're working closely with our coaching clients, that we can't expect to lead a positive life when we have a negative attitude.

We can't control what we think, but what we can do is control how we react to our thoughts and that is why we have such a strong push towards doing these daily rituals.

So we can alter how we think first thing, which leads to how we feel and then how we act rather than just reacting to our thoughts. Remember that there will always be things about a situation that we can control, even if the only thing we can control is our thoughts and actions and attitude towards them. Sometimes it may mean digging a little bit below the surface to find them.

We're going to quickly overlook two key mindsets which we feel we can categorise a majority of people into, the first one being a fixed mindset.

This is where a person has a mindset that can limit their potential to achieve their goals. They will accept their basic qualities for being them, and they don't really improve them too much. They are reluctant and often very resistant to change

These are the kinds of people that really need to work on their mindset even more, to learn and understand how they can train their brain to accept that they can improve. It is possible for them to strive towards being the best version of themselves, whatever that means to them.

Now we've come onto the growth mindset. This is where we start to understand that our basic abilities and qualities are just the starting point, and they're a starting point for us to build upon and learn more and to develop ourselves and work towards the best version of ourselves, our goals and beyond.

So if you don't naturally have this mindset, we need to work a little harder to embody a growth mindset, so it becomes a lot more consistent towards progress and what the best version of you really is.

Only once you have that, will you ever reach your goals, if they are big goals, which if they're not, we want to work on that too. This is why we strive towards getting that mindset in before we work on anything else, because that mindset is what will get you started, that mindset is what will tell you, you can achieve your goals, you can begin to feel better about yourself, you can like what you see in the mirror, and, that's what this is all about.

The brain is just like a muscle. It needs to be trained or conditioned. That conditioning will keep you working towards and aligned with your goals even when internal resistance kicks in and even other 'life' factors could normally derail you.

We are strong believers in the way we think will affect the results we get. If we can think positively and adopt the right mindset, we will get the right results, like we said you get what you focus on.

For example, when it comes to body goals 80% of the people we have worked with have this trend that it's not really about diet and exercise, but even when they know this, they will focus on just that. The same when it comes to career, it's not really about the environment or about the job itself. It's about the mindset , they know this, yet still look to change their job or focus on the physical environment rather than the mindset. This is why we simply must address mindset right from the offset, so you hit the ground running

When first looking at mindset, we like to take a bird's eye view of your life and its entirety. So by this, we mean taking a step out and removing your emotions from certain things and situations and looking into where you are right now, not literally but internally, where are you? Where your current mindset is, how you're now feeling, and how important things in your life are to you.

Once you take this bird's eye view perspective of your life, you can make more rational decisions and train yourself to think better so you become closer, both physically and emotionally to those goals that are so important to you. You will remove yourself from doing things that are less important to you. Only when you do that, you will then have the time, energy, and commitment towards those valuable goals of yours.

Let us ask you a question, when was the last time you just stopped for a second and looked at the world going on and asked yourself, how am I today? Am I happy?

When you look into your mindset, you need to remove your ego, that won't help you. Remove any thoughts about yourself and really look deep, begin to question everything.

Look below the surface and you almost have to get comfortable being uncomfortable because you need to question your thoughts and the things you would normally accept for being true, as these thoughts have got you to here, where you are now. To progress in all areas of our life, we need to acknowledge some form of internal change is necessary.

Now, let's just say right here, now, it's not saying that what you've been thinking and what you've been feeling isn't right, however, what you've been thinking and what you've been feeling could possibly slow your ability to make that life-changing progress.

That's why we need an approach that really does focus that mindset. We need to do the work and learn more about ourselves and what's really important to us **and 'the why'** **it's important to you..**

The why it's important.

The why you want it -- the why now.

Because we all know it will get uncomfortable. Therefore, we need something that will keep us moving forwards when it is uncomfortable to stop us from throwing the towel in and being another story of not achieving your goals.

We are strong believers that anything that happens in our life has an effect on us. Things that happen to us physically and emotionally will have an effect on us and then on how we react to things, both immediately and in the future.

So you have struggled with committing to your goals and seeing them through until you've achieved them, there's a reason you struggle with this. There's a reason you can't get to where you want to be, and more importantly, stay there and before we go into this we want you to know that, you are not alone with the feelings you currently have but our aim is to show you a clear path to being the best version of yourself healthily and sustainably.

There could be an emotional attachment to food, it could be stress, anxiety, fear of failure, it could be many reasons. That's why we think it's important for you to address the underlying issue as to why you're not where you want to be before you go on

Once you question why you're not yet where you want to be in all of the 4Bs you can begin to truly move forwards. Self-awareness is key for longer term success. When we make significant progress in our mindset and only when, can we then move forward and achieve sustainable results with our Besties, Body, Brain, and Business. However, only once we have complete self-awareness, can you really start to create long-term change.

Now, this is something that both of us found a bit hard to understand and get to grips with when we first adopted these principles. However, traveling to the states twice to learn more on this topic, we found that many of the people who were doing well and were what we deemed successful had various daily rituals that they claimed helped them achieve success. We then felt it was really important that we adopt our own daily rituals to help us and show our clients this too.,

Over the years, since we started getting our clients doing this and doing this ourselves (we do practice what we preach), the results that they have seen have been dramatically better. Both physically and perhaps more importantly mentally, they've felt the benefits of their progress emotionally, which then means their loved ones all benefit from a happier, healthier version of them.

OK, we will put this another way for you now. When you begin to put your mindset first and begin daily rituals, everyone around you gets a happier and healthier you.

It's important before we get started on our journey physically to recognise that we need to take the time to create a goal that is important to you in all 4 areas of your life. An idea for you, if you like, specific to you and what you really want. This process is to create your own vision, a vision you can hold onto, even when you perhaps feel like giving up.

We find that having visions both long term and short term makes it much easier for you to get into the right mindset for working towards them. You take the time to feel the moment, live in that moment when those goals have been achieved.

You want to see it, you want to feel it, and you want to have all your emotions associated with it so that that invigorates immense passion about achieving your goals before you start your daily rituals. How would achieving your goals change your life for the better?

Then when we start the daily rituals, you're primed because you really want it. You know what it feels like and you know what it looks like.

So, now for some work to do, every day, you want to write out your goals. However, this isn't just jotting them down, it's emotionally connecting with them pen to paper (we did say to do this by pen? Your brain is connected to your thumb) The first thing you do, every single day, if you're running late, 2 minutes won't make it any worse.

If you don't have time because mornings are busy (yes, we hear you saying that as you shake your head)…

Get up 5 minutes earlier, this is VERY important. This is the most valuable 5 minutes of your day. .

Then we need to list three things you will do today to move forward. Now it doesn't need to be a massive jump, it could just be a small step in the right direction, as simple as reducing my portion size or as simple as I will walk to work today and even that you will not talk negatively about yourself today or I will send that email I've been putting off. Basically, things that will contribute to your goals. It doesn't need to be perfect. It's just progress that we're after.

A question we use to help find these little steps is-
What will make today a good day?

Daily Gratitude - change your perspective

SINCE WE STARTED Daily Gratitude, it has literally transformed our lives. Ok, maybe you're thinking, these guys say a lot of things have changed their life, but the truth is many of the things we cover in this book have. We couldn't be writing this book without it.

We have to admit before we did it, we thought it was a waste of time. We thought it was something we could do more productively like many do, for example, watching the soaps on TV. However, we persevered with it, spend five minutes every day getting ourselves into a state of gratitude, and we've never looked back. In fact, any time we feel sad, miserable or just generally like everything is against us, we know we simply aren't seeing the things we have to be grateful for.

Because when you are in a complete state of gratitude, you begin to realize a lot of what we stress about isn't overly important. We stress about things beyond our control, and that takes our focus away from what's right in front of us.

After months of practicing gratitude daily and seeing how it positively impacted our bodies, brains, besties and business, we preached it to our clients, and they've also found the exact same thing. How much of a difference spending that few minutes a day every day being **truly, genuinely** grateful for things has made to their life. Less stress, more happiness, in a nutshell.

How often do you do it ,just drift from one day to the next, doing your thing without sitting there and appreciating how far you've come. Answer this, when was the last time you just sat there and looked at some of the things in life you have to be grateful for? Not anytime recently if you're like most. Like we said, we don't judge.

Yes, you may still have quite a journey ahead of you. That's still cool, however, you do need to take time to appreciate how far you've come too. You've got this far, you've done some work already. Even if it's just being grateful for getting this book and starting your journey to long term health and happiness from today, that's something to be grateful for.

Let's be honest here, when was the last time you cleared your mind and sat in the moment and were totally grateful?

This will help you recognise that there are ALWAYS things to be grateful for, and by doing this you'll be able to approach many of 'life's challenges' with a new perspective that says 'things may not be ideal but I always have things to be grateful for'. In fact, this is something that changed the game for Elly who used to struggle to sleep but practicing this helped her focus on the positives that are always there.

If you're somebody who's naturally a negative thinker or perhaps somebody who naturally has a closed mindset, it's even more vital you take the time to do these daily rituals in order to change that mindset over time.

Here we like to use the trip advisor example to show that it is normal to focus on the negative things, so we have to work hard to change that focus. Like how many times when you go on trip advisor or other review sites when looking at things, are you drawn to and put off by the negative reviews? Like there could be hundreds or even thousands of positives but someone didn't like the decor in the bar area or something else that previously wouldn't have concerned you but now? You let their 1 star rating put you off? It is common that negatives can hold more weight in our mind. This is going to require some serious training to adapt to the focus point.

Please, please, please, don't think this will happen overnight, okay! It's just like the whole process of becoming the best version of yourself.... this takes time, you are here and to get there, there's a process which with all the will in the world cannot and should not be rushed. In fact adopting a mindset that's completely aligned with your goals can take a lifetime, in fact many people never truly do it. They just drift and settle for less than they really want. Because 'life'. However, if you choose to invest in your mindset so it leads you where you want to go, it might mean we take a little bit longer to perhaps notice the physical progress on this journey, but the emotional progress will be tenfold.

You must not rush this process, take time on it and it saves you a lot of time, frustration, and heartache in the long run. We are sure you have heard the saying before, the quick fix is not really the quick fix?

Personal Development is a very, very important part of the mindset, because we know if we don't develop our mind, we can never truly develop as a person physically, either. That's why we spend at least ten minutes each day on what we like to call personal development. Remember we are talking baby steps daily not hammering it for a few hours a day then a week later, forgetting everything. A few minutes each day CONSISTENTLY.

So part of doing this personal development, could be to spend five to ten minutes every day reading or watching videos or listening to podcasts, usually on mindset, or self-help but could be something relating to your career goal or your relationship goals, basically we want to work on developing your knowledge area that will help you get closer to your goals every single day. So we read, watch or listen until we get at least one point that we can take away and reflect on it, even if it's just a few minutes. Since we started implementing this in our programs our clients have noticed a shift too.

We know many people who are kings/queens of reading, they will read a book in a day, ask them what they learnt, very few can answer, ask them what they implemented, even less can answer that. So that's why we only want to take one thing away that we can implement or properly learn.

So, invest ten minutes each day on personal development and we can promise you the rewards will be well worth it. Even if it means you get up ten minutes earlier. Those ten minutes, you see, won't make much of a difference as that personal development will.

POSITIVE AFFIRMATIONS/COMMITMENTS

One thing we can always rely on to make ourselves have a quick shift in mindset is positive affirmations/commitments. When we start to feel like we are stressed out, pent up, frustrated, annoyed, it is always good to take a step back and start with doing either some positive affirmations or positive commitments.

Ryan, Elly what is the difference between them? You ask. Well it's a subtle difference but one will suit some more than others. Affirmations are often making positive statements about yourself often in the present tense. This will shift the mind, for example- I am a strong man/woman and I can get through this. Which is great and can really help however if you're a negatively tuned person you may have that little voice inside your head that is like 'no, you can't, who are you kidding?'. Trick is, you need to believe what you are saying.

Many of our clients see great success with affirmations, as does Elly, whereas Ryan is known to have more of a negative view that does seem to instill that doubt so positive commitments are more suited to him. Really which one works for you will be purely down to you, however, you have to believe it, so there's no point going through the motions on this, in fact anything mindset related, should not be a case of boxing ticking it's very much a case of getting emotionally connected to the goals.

It's important to take time to sit down and either find the positives which are there after some digging, or making them positive commitments to look forward to achieving the,. Because let's face it, it is easy to get drawn up and hung up upon those negative or bad things that happen within your life and your lifestyle because they will always be there.

However, once you start to shift that focus to a more positive thing we can build on that. Remember, we aren't saying ignore the negative things, but we don't want to dwell on them and be your only focus.

A way to look at it is, treat and talk to yourself the way you would talk to your best friend. Say they're being hard on themselves about their body shape, their role as a parent, their career, you'd probably be looking around to help them focus on positive things. This is where we tell you to **take your own advice #NotSorry** So take that time if you feel like you're running around stressed out, fed up and everything feels negative and you can slip off the wagon, this is your time to do these positive affirmations.

Again, a bit of bad news, It will feel uncomfortable the first couple of times you do it because often we are conditioned to be negative or hard on ourselves, but once we make this a habit we can guarantee you it will be the best thing you've ever done.

Positive affirmations and commitments have changed the lives of both of us and our clients over the last 5 years since we started practicing them.

LIFESTYLE

IF YOU ARE on a journey of personal development of any kind, it can make socialising more of a challenge. Often self-progress and socialising don't come together. Which can often mean people wanting to make progress with their personal goals, particularly with their body and their brain and their business goals, feel the need to avoid all social situations all together. However we are here to tell you, that, if the journey you are on is promoting this, you need a change of approach as this is not sustainable for you and your plan is wrong, no ifs, no buts, yes even if you think 'but if i just knuckled down for now', **even you** need to have a leveled approach in order to feel happy and emotionally healthy.

We know that your goals are really important to you and you've got that constant reminder of why they're important to you because you're doing your daily rituals and you're constantly reminding yourself of your goals, what they are, and most importantly, how important they are to you.

This is when we move onto that lifestyle because, every single thing we do equates to or makes up what our lifestyle is. We have had an extremely hectic and poorly balanced lifestyle at times, working ridiculous amounts of hours when Ryan had Fit Body Jersey he was working 15+ hours a day, plus trying to fit both of our training sessions in, plus trying to find time for Aoife-Mae, it was chaotic, to say the least.

Elly had also worked in finance for 8 years where her lifestyle comprised feeling the guilt of not at work by 8 am, most days working through her lunch break, grabbing what she could when she could have the convenience of the chocolates left by colleagues were an easier choice especially when workloads were high during this time she did not see the benefits to taking a time out even if it was for just 15 minutes as this would even benefit her work productivity. Elly will also admit that confusion about what she could eat made it a lot more difficult to make healthier choices.

Sleep became a nice-to-do rather than a necessity, and eating well was something that really slipped too, all because our lifestyle was so poorly balanced. We opted for convenience over importance and health and we felt

- ✔ Tired
- ✔ Fed up
- ✔ Lethargic

And if we had carried it on and not decided we needed to change, not only would we have suffered, but Aoife-Mae would have too.

That's why we want you to focus on getting that balance around your lifestyle so that things become more sustainable. So what is a balanced lifestyle? It's an important question and we would say you could ask 100 people and get 100 different answers, but to us, *a balanced lifestyle is living a happy and healthy life that helps you deliver the results in all areas of your life according to the importance they hold to you.*

That being said it must also be sustainable, which if you've come this far into the book, you will know is of high importance to everything we talk about by now.

So by that we mean you aren't depriving your health, you aren't depriving your family, you really aren't depriving your work and you certainly aren't depriving yourself, oh and there's social time too (unless you're as boring as us).

That is why we want you to focus on getting that mindset right before you move on to this lifestyle part. If you haven't got the mind in the right place, forget this, go back and read the mindset chapter again and get to establishing those goals and why they're important again.

Once you've done that, continue reading.

Whether you like it or not, everything should be around your specific lifestyle and what works for you long term. We often say to clients if you can't sustain it, don't start it. We've seen it all too often since joining the 'fitness industry'. People setting themselves goals, start a new plan, a journey to recreate themselves and try to change their lifestyle overnight.

Then a few months later they're wondering why the progress has been temporary. Why they can't sustain the results, they wonder why they cannot sustain that 'new' lifestyle that almost brushed everything that was already in their life to the side. Then they feel like crap a few months later when they realise they're now even further away from where they were beforehand.

However, they have no one but themselves to blame because they got a plan that wasn't sustainable for them..

You may have experienced this when focusing on your career, you work later, focus on studying at the weekend and miss out on social times with family, or perhaps with your weight loss goals you're out for a meal with friends and you are there having a salad with no dressing and sparkling water.

Let us break this to you, no happy night out started with a salad without dressing and a sparkling water (unless of course you genuinely love that).

Everything with the above approaches were temporary. We find this only leads to resentment of what you are doing, there is no enjoyment factor which means adherence to the plan is low, again another way to make us feel low because we have not stuck to something we said we were going to.

What we do with all of our coaching clients is work on getting the mindset right and recognising how important your goals are. Then, we look at getting that lifestyle in place and seeing how we can adapt to their current lifestyle.

We'll say again - **we adapt their current lifestyle to make progress** (wow we made it bold too) and only then do we look at nutrition and exercise. Everything is around exactly what you're doing now and tweaking it and improving it so that when you make that progress, the progress is there to stay, whether it be weight loss, career progress, or even relationship progress because anything you've done is sustainable.

Like, answer these questions, who wants to progress their career but lose their relationships? Who wants to be in good shape but boring and miserable? Answers on the postcard ☺.

When you talk about lifestyle, it's all about choices and priorities. It's survival first, right? There are some necessities in life versus some things that could be called 'our nice to-dos.' And we often find that things like working out and trying to be really strict with your diet are nice to-dos rather than necessities and even as health and fitness coaches helping people be that best version of themselves we would 100% agree with it – necessities aren't training and diet, they really aren't.

Necessities are things like, looking after the kids, getting the housework done, going to work. These are things that you need to do day to day. That's why you need to make sure that everything you're doing works around your necessities and lifestyle, rather than doing it the opposite way around.

We've lost count in the number of times we've come into contact with potential clients or clients that have unfortunately done it the opposite way around and found that the other areas of their life have struggled, and the necessities aren't being done, but the nice to dos are for a period of time which at the time seems ok until, the house is a tip and you have no clean clothes for work, the kids are hungry, or being affected because you're focused so hard on them other areas, and you are on a final warning at work for either being late all the time or uniform not being clean (you get the picture right?).

However, if you've done this, give it a few weeks and actually take a step back and notice how many things in your life aren't being done that realistically, you know should be getting done.

It can become very frustrating and make you resent working towards your goals, and this is the last thing we want. After all, what's the point in working towards a goal? One thing's for sure, it's not resenting it? It should make us excited knowing we are working to better ourselves, opportunity to live our best life.

You should look forward to it and the life that is actually making that progress to your life will achieve or create. You should enjoy it. This is an experience or journey that, hopefully, you will live with for a long time.

To put it in perspective, we have worked with top corporates who we think 'oh wow, they have the life' only to find out when we delve a bit deeper, they're working super long hours, struggling to get finished to read their kid a bedtime story, or can't have dinner as a family. That is totally fine for some but it's an understandable sacrifice some have made.

Like that fitness model on the cover of a magazine, they look great for the photo, but they've dieted for 16 weeks, perhaps missed their best friend's big birthday party and haven't had a meal with their family where they all eat the same food for months, for a photoshoot? Still want that body shape?

So we aren't saying for a second everyone who is successful in a particular area has had to miss out on another area but it's easily done by many and seen as a price to be paid for the success they see in a particular area. However, we know with this lifestyle-based approach you CAN and SHOULD feel success in all areas. We feel we have achieved it and maintained it for the last 5 years now.

So have a look around, next time you see that person who's where you want to be, what do they do on a day-to-day basis? What is their lifestyle like? Are they more active than you? Are they following a different path than you? Can you see the bigger picture, rather than just the athletic body shape, successful career or really big social circle or whatever you deem as successful? These are questions that are worth asking yourself in order for you to accept and realise how important lifestyle really is and then realise if what you think you want, is actually what you want.

Total Transparency here:- We, for example, would love to walk around like those models you see on the front of fitness magazines, however knowing the strict diets, harsh training regimes and cardio sessions they will have to commit to, we know we don't really want it. We enjoy having ice cream with our girls or pizza with lots of wine to wash it down. So we settle for a shape we can be happy with whilst enjoying that lifestyle where pizza and wine is involved too.

Once you see this and recognise that to get where you want to it may require significant change, please do not rush these changes, take it one step at a time, and remember it's a process and one that takes time.

If you're trying to change your lifestyle and you have children, it becomes even more important to address it as a whole lifestyle, because we all know our children learn from us.

Our children pick up our habits from us, children will adopt those habits and they can stay with them even later on in life. So if you're hopping from diet to diet, exercise fad to exercise fad, or even career path to career path your children will learn from that and your children are likely to adopt the very same mentality towards, well, life! SO consider this question before you go on that pursuit of your goals, would you be happy with your children following the same path?

We both noticed this when we were prepping for a bodybuilding show in September 2016. Our eating habits had changed significantly, as they needed to in order to get 'show ready' and we ate little food that we usually did (again the results we achieved were temporary). Then Aoife-Mae became fussy and a bit of a nightmare for food this was a real wake up call for us as her role model, because as parents we are our children's first role models in life. We realised in that moment we had to change not just for us but the future of our daughter. We want her to live a life filled with health and happiness therefore it is up to us to show her the way starting with our own actions. Now we have Niamh too so it is so important we show the girls this lifestyle approach, so that they'll see mummy and daddy living a lifestyle that delivers success across all areas of their life. As opposed to them seeing a parent with success in one area but missing out on others.

When you take the time to look at lifestyle, it's important to recognise sometimes it's not just about doing more, for example, if you want to progress your career, it doesn't necessarily mean you need to work harder, or even longer, perhaps just working smarter with a clear path?

When wanting to lose weight it doesn't mean needing to exercise more it could just mean being smarter with activity and your calorie intake? As we guess, right now, you're probably pretty busy, right? This is where so many people fall down,trying to add more or should we say MORE to their already busy life.

Leading to the next question, are you sleeping okay? Sleep has a massive impact on our ability to perform. If you're not sleeping right, your body will not function to its best, therefore we cannot expect to see the progress we want if we are sacrificing our sleep. We read a book a few years back called Essentialism by Greg McKewon where he describes sleep as your asset.

When you think of it like this, you want to grow your assets or protect them right? The same should be said for sleep. We have found with many clients when we have helped them to implement some simple changes to their lifestyle to give them an extra hour of sleep, the physical results have improved, even when we changed nothing else, but what's even more important? The emotional progress they found from this too. Often finding they're about to put more into things and everyone around them benefits. So never underestimate the importance of sleep. It really is your asset. Sleeping patterns are part of your lifestyle.

SLEEP

SLEEP IS possibly one of the most important aspects of high performance. Now before we go on, we aren't just talking high performance in work, or at sports like many associate it with, we are talking day to day living your best life and becoming the best YOU. It's also probably the most boring part and the most commonsense part. However, you'd be surprised how little people sleep when they're trying to work towards goals that perhaps they feel are tough to achieve. The thought of 'oh, I can create an extra hour or two a day (by sleeping less) I will get more done'. But it rarely works like this. In fact, when we first started Hodgson Health we did it around being booked PTs, having a baby, Ryan had 2 businesses with staff, 4 locations and well was busy. We tried the whole less sleep thing to get stuff done, but we found the quality and efficiency of the work we did took a dive and we ended up spending twice as long correcting things and improving on them. So for you to be your best you need to prioritise your sleep.

Again, as always, we sound like a broken record with this but we do 'get it.' Because you're already busy and then you try to throw in things such as journaling, reading, committing to goals, oh and diet and exercise that all takes a little bit more out of your day, sometimes it can be tempting to set that alarm a little earlier, which can be fine but then if you pair it with the 'I've not done everything yet I need to stay up later' and think fuck it, I will just catch up on sleep another time. It can be a recipe for disaster.

However, sleep is just as important as everything else if not more important. We don't need to explain to you how important sleep is in too much of an in-depth scientific way. But we want you to remember that when you go to sleep, your body is getting that recovery and that rest it needs to get everything in the right place, from the recovery of the cells in the body to get your hormones in the right balance. So you can do everything at your best.

We suggest getting a minimum of six hours of sleep. Ideally, you want to be aiming for eight hours. Yes, people can survive on less.

Yes, you might feel okay on less. However, we would bet you any money you'll feel better hitting more towards that 6-8 hours.

Often the more you sleep, the more you feel you need it but that's just because your body is getting more finely tuned and it's recognising that it needs sleep. It's like we speak to many busy parents surviving less than 6 hours and saying they feel ok, but it's simply what they've become accustomed to. Forget the importance of sleep and let other things take priority then, you'll probably start to form a habit of sleeping less and less.

Are you stressed? Again stress has a negative impact on your body's ability to adapt both physically and mentally towards a healthier lifestyle. Cortisol levels when that high, affect everything from digestion to sleep to moods. When we are stressed, we simply cannot expect to get the best results, physically or emotionally.

These are some of the biggest factors of lifestyle that can really make a difference towards becoming the best version of you. However, we do think there are several tools or steps you can take to increase activity levels in your lifestyle, without having to dramatically 'do more', which we do find is a common belief from people starting out on their journey to self-progress, because we know doing more is not always the answer, in fact doing less but better is often the answer. We often don't have the time to do more, because let's face it, say you finish reading this book and you set goals with your 4Bs (which we hope you will) , the rest of your life doesn't stop. Also, we like to talk a lot about being parents because well, life is busy and whatever you're doing is being watched by them and we think you'll agree with us when we say that only if we can be a good role model to our children, will they lead a happy, healthy, fit life.

When you're looking at the lifestyle we suggest you take a look around at those people who are possibly where you want to be or are in the shape you would like to have, we have this saying we follow and it's 'success leaves you clues'.

We got this from our first online coaching mentor AJ Mihrzad. By this, it means if you look at the lifestyle that those people are leading, what they do from day to day, the lifestyle they're leading will leave clues for you on how to get into that place both physically and emotionally.

So, when you look at diet and exercise further on in this book, you can see that those people who are perhaps in shape may follow a particular diet that won't work for you and your unique challenges.

They may even follow a particular activity/ training regime that will not fit your unique lifestyle challenges. It's the same with that high flying director with a great career. They may be able to do more to commit to it than your current lifestyle allows.

So really, take time to look at the bigger picture of what you really want vs. what they actually have, so look at their 4Bs take some clues but be aware you may not actually want what these previously seemingly successful people have. We have seen this when it comes to the body shapes we look to, then we often see those with the body we may desire, whether it is a female Elly aspires to be like or a male Ryan does, they may not have 2 kids, be able to enjoy a glass, ok a bottle, of wine on the weekend and so on. **Think Bigger Picture.**

Their lifestyle will be something that is revolved around them and what really works for them because they too have their unique challenges, to achieve that body, brain besties and/or business. For them to maintain it, they're following a lifestyle that allows it.

So remember that success leaves clues.

Follow the people that are successful and learn from them because that's all we've done. Now we don't like to call ourselves a success as such but we literally coach our clients on what we do, because it works every time it's followed.

We're just two parents who are working hard to try to help more people to feel better about themselves and become the best version of themselves, and we work on being the best version of ourselves, within that is a lifestyle and a lot of clues that you can take away.

Note, it's not copying another person's lifestyle as it won't work for you, it's a case of looking at the things they do and seeing if you can implement some of these things into your daily life.

We don't have a magic gift. All we want to do is deliver our message and by doing so we help you understand that success leaves clues and you can learn a lot by following the footsteps of those who are perhaps further ahead on their journey in an area than you.

Now, going in a little more into the lifestyle, it's where we talk about a 'priorities list' as you are now sort of leveling out your whole life seriously, you'll account for every second.

So, what we do is list all the things you need to do on a day-to-day basis or all the things you feel should do in your day, not right now, but to get where you want to be.

Then, we begin to prioritise.

We begin to put the things we have to do. For example, we have to go to work so we can afford to live; we have to make food for the children, etc.

Then, we look at the nice-to-dos or the things we probably spend more time doing than we need to do and once we start to limit those, we can dedicate more time towards having a happy, healthy, balanced lifestyle because that's what we're aiming for here.

Everything needs to fit into your lifestyle, not the lifestyle needs to fit into everything else. Which by this it is specific to you, just because it fits into your best friends doesn't mean it will fit into yours.

We often get told by new clients they have time to do things like, journal, exercise, or study to progress their career. However, taking time to do this we begin to find out, how much time they spend, scrolling their social media, running around after everyone else, not being as productive as they would like. They almost create hours each week within 30minutes. So **invest** time to do this activity.

Map your week out and put in the non-negotiables, then the other bits around it, based on your priorities. Like don't say you want to lose weight, don't have time to exercise but you spend 3 hours a week watching TV (most people spend more than that, but it's just an example).

Once we've got that ingrained into our brain, we can really take control of our lifestyle and the progress we are looking to make. We talk about balance time and time again throughout this book because we cannot emphasise enough the power of having a well-balanced lifestyle. But again, don't forget, that balance needs to be right for you and only you, no one else.

Once you've got that right for you, and everyone else works on themselves, everything will just fall into place.

As you've already read so far, we are huge on planning. We recommend the more you plan, the better results you will get in all areas of your life.

If you can plan every single detail of your day, your week, your month, your year, you will be a lot more likely to achieve your goals in fact of the 1,000s of women we have helped the one thing we notice that really hits home on the difference between, ok to great results, is planning.

You'll feel more committed because you've planned it. Yes, we know sometimes life gets in the way, of course, it does, and that's where even if you've got your commitment levels and the mindset right, you'll have a backup plan or the right mindset that won't allow you to give up or throw in the towel, you'll just work around the hiccups that life has thrown at you.

We find taking time on a Sunday evening when most people would relax and perhaps forget about what's about to start, i.e. the week that's about to start. So spending half an hour (even less sometimes) planning your week out can make a big difference.

Almost everyone dreads that Monday feeling and we find that planning on that Sunday for the week, so you know what to expect for the week, and you are in control of it, physically and emotionally.

This will relieve a massive amount of stress and pressure on you going into the new week. You can also see how once you've written it down and you've got a 'timetable' of some sort planned out, you can factor everything else around it because you've already got that in your diary. You've already got that in your planner, and then all you have to do is stick to the plan. By having the plan it'll increase your commitment towards it too. It is also worth mentioning that we have had clients who follow this and actually save money (and time and energy too)this way too.

The plan-

So now, every Sunday, you will map your week out from 12 am-11.59 pm. Including:

- sleep
- housework
- running around after the kids
- meals
- travel time
- family/friends time

☐ exercise

☐ studying

☐ Social life

☐ reading (*The Best Version of You, REVISED EDITION with the Hodgsons*)

You name it. If you do it, it goes in 'the plan.' Then, all you have to do is follow the plan. Now one thing we find by doing this with clients, they realise how much time they waste.

So don't be surprised if this happens, but this time is the time you can use to focus on you, your goals and what you want to achieve.

We always say when making a 'plan' or general weekly map it's important to try and make it as within your control as possible, by this we mean, trying not to rely on other people where possible. We find when you rely on others it can make it much more challenging and they may not understand the importance of your goals. Now it probably sounds kind of difficult, but the amount of people who will do things when they're trying to arrange childcare, they're trying to arrange different things to make sure they can do the various elements they feel they need to do to get into their life in order to work towards those goals..

However, as soon as you have to rely on somebody else, you're setting yourself up to possibly be let down. It's only when you start to remove relying on anyone else you can be certain you can move forwards.

So that's why if you need to arrange childcare to go to the gym, perhaps going to the gym isn't what you need right now. Now is not the time to use the gym. Perhaps just going out and being active with the children could be a good way for you to be active.

If you need to have somebody watch the kids while you prepare complex meals, you do not need to be making complex meals. You just need simplicity and things that can take a minimal amount of prep work.

If you need someone to help you with work to fit in the study, perhaps now isn't the time to study, you get our drift? It's as simple as that, breaking it down and looking at how much you can do yourself and how little you have to rely on others to move forward in any of them goals. The less you have to rely on others, the more it's on you and only you to work to move forward. Another thing with Lifestyle, when we talk to clients about it, they often think they need to go from being completely sedentary to being extremely active and burning loads and loads of calories.

However, this isn't the case.

Lifestyle incorporates literally everything, and it includes activity levels, it includes work, it includes family, it includes nutrition and it includes mindset **literally everything you do in your life is part of your lifestyle**.

Things to consider are: you don't necessarily need to be doing more exercise when it comes to making a more active lifestyle as such. For example, to be more active in life, you don't need to do more workouts or try to plan your day around going for runs or walks or to the gym.

It could be as simple as parking your car on the top floor of a multi-story car park and using the stairs to go up and down them. You've increased your step count, thus being more active.

Parking the car slightly further away in the car park, so you've got to walk further to get to work or to wherever you need to go. You've slightly increased your step count.

All of these steps start to add up and those steps equal more activity and calories burned.

Another way could also be to walk or cycle to work one or two days a week if it works around your lifestyle. That's what's really important because everything needs to fit around you and your lifestyle and what will work.

Let's just look for ways you can look at slight improvements. Just like we discussed on the mindset. Think of making even 1% improvement each day, these little bits of improvement add up.

Focus less on what you can't do and more on what you can do. We say if you struggle to find time to go to do things like going to the gym now, chances are even when you get into your regime, it will get in the way and something will end up having to give.

So start it the right way, the sustainable way that fits your lifestyle.

ELLY & RYAN HODGSON

OH, THE STRESS.

NOW, WHEN WE first established the importance of stress would be in this book, it was difficult for us to decide what area of the book to put this in because we think it could have fitted into the mindset section, however, we felt that based on the Western world lifestyle, it would sit better into the lifestyle, perhaps you'd describe your lifestyle as stressful? When we ask people to describe their lifestyle in a word, hectic is usually first, followed closely by stressful.

Because we know we often think about physical benefits to working towards goals in all areas, such as losing weight or toning up, having stronger relationships, earning more money etc. However, the psychological benefits can often outweigh those physical benefits longer term.

We know high levels of stress and even depression can really impact physical progress and overall levels of happiness and health. This is why we want you to try to create a low-stress lifestyle.

By doing that, ultimately, we need balance (yes, again that). Balance in your lifestyle you're not dedicating too much time to certain areas of your life and forgetting about others that will create stress because it's a vicious cycle. That's why you NEED the plan you made before, you did make a plan, right?

The cycle of stress is something that's very difficult to get out of and it's often something that's swept under the carpet by people and disregarded because they'll question themselves about what they have to feel stressed about or what they have got to feel worried about. But ultimately, we cannot control how we feel, but what we can do is put things in place to stop us from getting to that stage in the long-term.

Questioning your thoughts surrounding stress is a really good tool to use.

HOW MUCH DO YOU DESERVE IT?

A question that is always worth asking yourself is how much you deserve to achieve your goals. Like given the level of effort and commitment you've put into achieving them, how much do you really deserve it?

. Now that's based on your lifestyle, based on your mindset, and based on everything, all folded into one.

Because if you think you're just going to get them without working for it, you're wrong, unfortunately, of course, we have made this book to make it as accessible as possible, however, it doesn't mean it's easy.

Now we know that everywhere you look now there are 'quick fix' options being marketed to you left right and centre, lose 3 stone in a month, earn 6 figures in 6 weeks, find true love in a week, and so on. It's all about a quick fix, there's very little talk about playing the long game, seeking consistency and looking at the long game.

The reality is you have to work, you will have to make changes. As you've already established in the first two parts to this book, when we covered mindset and we went over lifestyle, **something has to change.**

Because doing what you're doing has got you where you are now. But to have self-progress, you want to move forward, you want to become the best version of yourself, you want to achieve your goals.

That is why it is vital you ask yourself the question: do I deserve the results? And if the answer is no, then you know what you've got to do; get that mindset right, get that lifestyle adapted, and then you'll make sure you deserve it. Only then you can feel hard done by if you don't achieve the results.

See, we live in a world where people will often spend more time trying to justify why they didn't achieve their goals, trying to conjure up excuses as to why someone is further ahead than them, than actually doing the work.

NUTRITION

SO NOW, we will move on to the third principle of becoming the best YOU. This is nutrition, we won't sugar coat it (see what we did there?). The hard work has already been done.

However, it's worth mentioning one key difference between now at the time of writing this book and when we wrote the original is the word we use. We use the word nutrition in a bid to avoid the word diet, as often when we call it our diet, people have the thought of it being temporary, whereas this is not temporary, remember we are thinking the long game, right?

That's right, this part now becomes the easier part, which we are guessing you would have focused on first-diet and exercise. But **these are only the easy parts after the Mindset and Lifestyle have been addressed.**

Now the reason it gets easier is that the nutrition and exercise will fall into place and the only reason it will fall into place is that you've spent the time to get your mindset right and spent the time to balance the lifestyle and make sure it's balanced in a way that works for you. If you haven't done that go back and re-read the first two steps again. Seriously, it may seem like a time-waster, but it's actually a time-saver in the long run. Think about it that quick fix you've tried several times over the years, was it really a quick fix?

When you look at nutrition, it's important to remember that one day, or one week, even one month of eating a well-balanced diet or following controlled nutrition guidelines does not make you healthy.

Just like one salad doesn't make you healthy, we also say one burger and chips or one pizza will not make you unhealthy or fat. It's important to remember, as we've already mentioned in this book, **we are a direct product of the lifestyle we've led up to now.**

So by this we mean, give yourself time to create a positive change, particularly for diet, because there will, yet again, be internal resistance.

Understand that it can take a little time to see sustainable progress, but once you do have that patience and you see the change, you'll be grateful for following this piece of advice for the rest of your life because you will not fear to have a burger and chips or a pizza or an ice cream or a bottle or two of wine.

You're also not going to dread the thought of having a salad every day for your dinner, because it will not happen if you do it the right way from the offset.

When you look on an online search engine, 'best diet to lose weight', there are literally thousands, if not millions, out there.

- ✔ High carb.
- ✔ Low carb.
- ✔ High fat.
- ✔ Low fat.
- ✔ Intermittent fasting.
- ✔ Renegade diet.

There are so many options out there when it comes to nutrition. So many ways they all promise you quick results in a safe, sustainable way that will make you feel great overnight.

And the reality is they all may work, to some degree.

They can all probably give you the physical results you're looking for the short term but,

It's all about one thing, IIFYL.

That means **If It Fits Your Lifestyle.**

So, we know if we can get your lifestyle correct, you can achieve great long-term results.

So, for some people, it might be intermittent fasting that works well (not eating for a 'fasting window' regularly). For others, it might be the renegade diet.

Then, go into more depth is about how you feel when you're eating certain foods. For some, low carbs work better, for others (most), high carbs work better. Another factor to look at is enjoyment because nutrition is a big part of socials and ultimately we should enjoy what we eat.

When embarking into the world of nutrition, it is all about finding what's right for you. **Tracking it and assessing it** so you know what's right for you and ultimately, listening to your body (super important).

You know your body better than anybody else does, including the experts. Yes, the experts can find scientific studies upon studies that are going to back up what they feel, but ultimately, there will also be another expert that will find contradictory studies that will go against exactly what the other person or study has suggested. All too often, contradictory to each other with their own theories, studies, and rationale to support their argument. In fact, it's no wonder people are so confused about nutrition.

So, keep an open mind when it comes to nutrition. Keep an open mind as to what's right for you, and listen to your body because if you're on a diet. You're feeling like crap, that diet isn't working, regardless of what physical results you're seeing, because we should all have the same one goal in mind, to feel better regardless of what your physical goals are. If you don't feel better, it's not working.

Like let's face it, our nutritional intake fuels all of our goals, from our body goals, besties, business and brain, it all needs the right nutritional intake to suit.

So we would say at least 80% of the clients we have worked with have experienced emotional eating, and some more often than now when they tell us about it, they feel embarrassed. They feel embarrassed telling us they resort to food when they're feeling emotional.

However, there's something you should know because we get it. In fact, we've both been known to eat emotionally on negative occasions and it is more common than you'd think, just perhaps a lot of the fitness world, don't like to share it, but if you look closely, you can see many of those 'super lean' people have some form of distorted eating. However, let's look at emotional eating and why it can be quite common. When you're a baby and you cry and you're upset and you need comforting, what's the first thing you're given?

Normally, milk or food.

That makes you feel better and unfortunately, that attachment to food doesn't leave easily, in fact,it can stay with some of us for a lifetime, like when you feel down, sad, or worked up? Do you ever habitually go to food? It can help us escape that negative emotion, however, when we eat like this the awareness has often left us. That's why we always say to people, don't feel embarrassed or don't feel bad if you emotionally eat just start to become aware of what you're eating and also what perhaps caused you to turn to food (the emotional trigger).

What you want to do is minimise it and limit it. So if we can control our emotions a little better, we won't turn to food. Because trying to stop the emotional attachment to food is a lot more difficult than it is to try to control your emotions in general. Sometimes dealing with the initial emotion (the trigger) we were feeling is hard and we get that, but it is important to stay in the moment and deal with really how you are feeling, understand why and what will help you feel better this is so we can reduce the emotional cycle of eating as it won't help you longer term and that initial problem will still be there but now you feel worse too., often guilt.

That's another reason we put such a strong emphasis on getting **the mindset right** before you do anything else because if your mindset is right, so will your emotional state be.

That's what we work with at Hodgson Health, 'Best YOU Coaching Programme' (which BTW you can get a 7 days FREE trial hodgsonhealth.com/trial) we always look at mindset first. It's all about getting the mind trained in order for you to be geared to your longer-term goals, in a position of power over yourself.

Without the mindset, unfortunately, any progress you see will probably be short-term. Sorry to be the bearer of bad news, but without it, these results will be short-lived, so emotional eating is often a mindset issue as opposed to a nutrition-related one.

When your mindset is right nutrition does become much easier. Then we need to get the lifestyle right as we've already gone into it. IIFYL: If it fits your lifestyle.

This is by far more important than you getting a fad diet into your mind. Which if you embark on a fad diet, the results will be a fad too.

If you want a long-term result, long-term success, you need to focus on that lifestyle, get the lifestyle right, and then we know everything else will fit around it.

Thse two things already running smoothly will mean that your exercise and nutrition will be a walk in the park.

Diet or nutrition would probably be the second thing most people would think of focusing on to be healthy. But if you noticed, we've actually left exercise to last because nutrition is by far more important than exercise or as we call it activity.

Often the reason people opt for addressing exercise before they go for the diet is because they'll see quicker results by doing the exercise and feel like they're doing more to achieve their goal. It's a modern-day approach in the pursuit of instant gratification, like you'll often see on social media, people are always chasing that instant gratification for more likes, more followers and more praise.

When we look at nutrition, having a little bit of patience can really go a long way (yes, patience again).

It's important to look at what you're doing, **track it, assess it, and adapt it** accordingly, and you're making small changes at a time.

That's right, small changes are all we want. Perhaps 1-2 things at a time for long term success and the ability to enjoy the whole process too.

It's important to remember if you are working out your foods and you change everything overnight, you don't really know which change really made a difference.

That's why we say take things slowly and really do have some patience. Once you have more patience, the results you'll see will be permanent and you'll actually know why you have achieved them. Not just from a physical aspect, but from how you'll feel, your moods, your energy levels and hormones etc. So start to become aware of these, really understand as much as you can about yourself.

We often hear the term 'cheat weekends', cheat meals or relaxed weekends for diet and people trying to follow a diet of some kind, whereby people are fantastic Monday to Friday, really strict and then let it go on a weekend.

Now, although we get it, If you've had a tough week, and you're busy, trying to be strict with the food, by the weekend, you just feel like relaxing a little.

However, there's something you should bear in mind.

When you want to get towards that goal of being the best version of yourself, do you want to do it forever and seven days a week, or do you just want it for a few days of the week?

This probably sounds like a stupid question, but it's a valid question because you need to stay committed with a balanced approach towards your goals seven days a week. Think like this often when people have the 'cheat day'/ or even 'cheat meal' mentality, they suffer from many negative symptoms after it-

- Guilt
- Bloating
- Slower digestion
- Tiredness
- Water retention

Yes, you can still be slightly more relaxed. However, there's no point in being fantastic with the food Monday through Friday, keeping to your healthy calorie deficit and over eating all weekend to undo the deficit and eating loads of junk on a Saturday and Sunday (remember calorie in vs. calorie out).

So what we do is, we're pretty well balanced with the tracking strict Monday through Friday. Then Saturday and Sunday, we follow the 80/20 principle where we're eating 80% foods perceived as good or healthy and 20% slightly more relaxed. And we might increase our portion sizes slightly. But that's all.

That way, we never feel like we're depriving ourselves because, remember, if you have to call something a cheat meal or a cheat weekend, it means you're on a diet. Which often leads to the distorted eating we see quite vividly within the fitness industry as a whole. Using the term cheat on anything to us shows a lack of respect for what you were doing.

So even during the week when you're being strict, you can still fit in your favourite foods. If you enjoy a chocolate bar, you can work that into your diet. For example, if you're following the 80-20 we suggest and you're eating 1600 calories to eat towards your goals, that would mean you could have 320Kcals a day from 'relaxed' foods, so to speak.

We often find that when clients start to do this and they track their food first, they often don't turn to said foods as much, it's what you'll probably realise by trying to do that is that you don't really love that chocolate bar as much as you thought. Many will often "fall off the wagon" because they have deprived themselves of foods they enjoy, so keep the foods in, become aware of your nutrition as a whole and you are more likely to adhere to it.

So we use this comment to get you really rocking and rolling
Stop looking for a new diet, and look to improve the one you have already have

You have probably already noticed that this book is not like most self-progress books you've read in the past because we absolutely understand that chocolate tastes nice. Ice cream tastes nice. An ice-cold glass of wine washes down a burger and chips better than sparkling water does.

We 100% understand it. That's why we think it's absolutely vital you don't feel you need to be on a diet. You don't need to feel you need to deprive yourself of your favourite foods. It's all about understanding a little more about nutrition so you can see long-term sustainable results and stop feeling like rubbish and having to avoid every single social situation because we've been through that.

We spent years avoiding social situations through fear of the effect it would have on our body or through fear of our friends thinking we're weird. Now we're in a position where we kind of enjoy a social situation, eat and drink what we want within moderation, and also, we never, never feel guilty for it because we know it's all about lifestyle.

Then, before that, our mindset.

And because if they're both tuned right, this part becomes easy.

We need to understand and know that avoidance is never the answer. So by this, we mean, if you have a favourite food that's perhaps perceived as unhealthy, or you like foods you know aren't healthy for you, you should never avoid them.

What you should do is just know of them, the nutrients they contain, and know of the portion size you can eat without making your nutritional balance fly off. Once you address portion size and get that under control, there are absolutely no reasons you have to avoid your favourite foods.

Have you ever told a child they can't do something?

The answer is probably yes. And we bet when you told them they couldn't do it, the first thing they wanted to do was that one thing you told them they couldn't do.

It's the exact same for food.

If you were told you have to avoid things like bread, pasta, which we often hear in the modern world of dieting, avoid this, avoid that, it's the first thing that the person on that diet is thinking about.

Once they decide that they've had enough of the diet, they'll probably binge and overeat on those types of food.

So before you move on, we can't stress enough to you that **there is no such thing as bad foods. There's just bad portion control** and just bad choices.

Have you ever heard the saying you can't out train a bad diet? Well, we believe it's 100% true, and only when you realise, and recognise it, we begin to see those sustainable results you want to keep.

When we're talking about nutrition, it's important to start as simple as we can. Therefore, that's why we always talk about **calories first.**

In fact, we would go out on a limb here and say, if you don't have the calories right for you and your goals, you have no right whatsoever to be worrying about anything else when it comes to nutrition. Even though we see many people hopping to the more complex parts of nutrition first.

Buying their clean food salads and their avocados and nuts and seeds without even considering the calories first.

It is important form the start to ensure you are eating the right number of calories specific to you. You can work this out by going to hodgsonhealth.com/macros (it's free), but it takes into consideration your lifestyle to give you your Total Daily Energy Expenditure or TDEE. Once you have the calories right and they're right for you, and only you. Then move onto macronutrients.

Macronutrients (also known as Macros) which are proteins, carbs and fats. They're called macros because the body uses them in large quantities and again, contrary to popular belief in the diet world, none of these are the enemy.

Once we've got the calories right and the macronutrients right this will be you 90% of the way there in many aspects of achieving your goals. After macros, look at micronutrients. So that is your vitamins and minerals.

But here's the reality: people don't get fat or overweight by not having enough vitamin C or by having too much vitamin B. Ultimately, it's calories and macros for general weight loss.

So ultimately, for generally living a happy healthy life when it comes to nutrition, there are just 3 things to worry about-

1- Calories
2- Macros
3- Micros

When we talk about nutrition, it's really important to remember we don't need to over complicate things. As soon as we try to complicate things we are making it harder for ourselves.

We're in a world where there's so much information out there, and a lot of it is conflicting with each other. But truth be told, for example, a majority of the weight loss methods and theories will all help you lose weight for one simple reason:

CALORIES

All of the 'cleansing' or 'detox' options will work because of micros. Neither of these are complex, they're simply just a method dressed up in a way to make it more appealing to you.

When we look at the third aspect being micros, we don't even need to stress a massive amount about it now, simply trying to get plenty of colours into your food and if you're open to it, which you should be get a good quality multivitamin (the multivitamin doesn't replace a balanced diet). Just with how much we know about vitamins and minerals in the western diet getting everything in can be tricky, so a multivitamin can sort of 'tick the boxes,' so to speak.

We really don't like the word diet because it automatically makes people think it's temporary, and often when we discuss the word diet, people think about more extreme measures rather than what it actually means- (as per google)

noun

1.

> The kinds of food that a person, animal, or community habitually eats.

This is why we've emphasised during this book; it is all about **a permanent solution,** not a temporary one. The word habit is even in the definition.

There are so many diets out there with very conflicting pieces of advice. One is telling you to have really low carbs another is telling you to have a high carb/low fat, you have another one telling you to drink shakes. We have even seen others are saying you need to look at your blood group, we could go on listing the various 'reasons' people have used for promoting their diet as the best. It's no wonder people are confused.

However, it's all about one thing: **if it fits your lifestyle,** as we've already spoken about if you're a sociable person, what is the point in being on a super strict diet that restricts your favourite food?

When you read through a majority of these 'health books' or 'weight loss' books, they'll give you advice such as, if you're craving chocolate, or something sweet, have a cube of dark chocolate, and that will curb your craving.

Are they serious?

We don't know about you, but if someone gave us a cube of dark chocolate instead of a bar of Galaxy Caramel, or a Snickers chocolate bar, we'd be absolutely gutted. In fact, we'd probably throw the cube of dark chocolate at them (ok, we don't really have anger issues but we wouldn't be willing to accept that as a long-term strategy for food intake). Never mind the fact that avoiding foods only promotes an already unhealthy relationship with food. Did you know dark chocolate is higher in calories too.

That's why we don't find this advice relatable. It is all about balance, so if you're somebody who craves that chocolate and you want a bit of chocolate, have it, track it, be aware of the nutritional values in it and enjoy it- guilt free..

It's just about balance and about portion control, remember one chocolate bar won't make you unhealthy or fat, just like one salad or quinoa and hummus bowl won't make you healthy.

Now we know there are some people that will read this, thinking they are all or nothing; if they have a little, they'll have a lot. But if you track it and you make conscious, healthy decisions, which we will help you to do in this book, you will not need to avoid it.

You should not need to avoid it. In fact, we'd argue if you still feel the need to avoid your favourite foods, you haven't done the work on your mindset correctly, you aren't in control, so go back to the mindset part of this book and get that under control, why are you reading this again? That's right 'them' goals.

Just like if you want a glass of wine, have a glass of wine. It doesn't need to turn into a bottle or two bottles. One glass of wine will not ruin your progress, provided you've kept a healthy balanced lifestyle, and you keep your mindset in the right place. Bear that in mind when we read on in this chapter.

Now let's go into a little more depth. Just remember this one thing and you can't go too far wrong.

A calorie is a calorie - No ifs, no buts, now we know some will try to argue about why calories aren't all equal but for you and us, 'normal people' calories are calories. They are equal. 500 kcals of fruit vs. 500kcals of takeaway food contain the same amount of energy, now there's no denying the 500 Kcals of fruit would make you feel better thus perhaps help you burn more calories.

To keep it as simple as possible, as all, we need to do is make sure that the calories are right and the calories are right for you, nobody else. That's right for you, not your mate at work, or your auntie, or anyone else, just right for you and your goals. Based on your lifestyle, age and gender. As mentioned, you can get this worked out for FREE at hodgsonhealth.com/macros it gives you an approximate goal based on you, but note it is approximate. So then you need to use the 3 step process, track, assess then adapt based on the progress (or lack of) but remember patience here.

You can then make small adaptations to monitor the progress, part of the reason why most fail with this part is they go to extremes, they don't see or feel the progress they wanted so they decide they need to go much harder on themselves.

The number of people we have come across who have gone to try Keto, or Vegan based diets in a bid to 'eat healthy' so much so they cut out foods they enjoy. Which in turn can really have a negative impact on their relationship with food, and their journey as a whole. Yes even if you have watched a popular documentary, just keep yourself informed with an open mind.

We are big fans of flexible dieting, which is what we coach our clients on. It's often a revelation to them when we say you don't have to cut out the alcohol, you don't even have to cut out the chocolate if you enjoy it.

It ultimately means we are open to eating anything as long as it's within our quota of allowed calories and nutrients a day, so we track the macronutrients (in case you forgot, these are protein, carbohydrate and fat)

We'll say it again: Macronutrients are needed in large quantities in the diet. That means we should not be cutting them out. We need to have a balance across all three. Therefore, always make sure you have proteins, carbs, and fats in your diet – whichever way you decide to go, some of all three will be in a well-balanced diet.

Now we will say there is no such thing as 'essential carbs' however, there are essential proteins (Essential Amino Acids) and fats (Essential Fatty Acids) however from a performance (in overall life), feel good and enjoyment perspective we would never suggest cutting out carbs. We've found clients who cut carbs, struggle with social occasions and generally don't enjoy it and what's the point in a diet or nutrition plan you don't enjoy?

There are a lot of fads out there that will often cut out either carbs or fats. However, this is not optimal for long-term sustainable results and ultimately lifestyle too. Ever been on a low carb diet trying to eat out?

You can lose a lot of weight quite quickly by going on a really low carbohydrate diet. Often, within a couple of weeks, you can lose 10 to 12 pounds. A majority of this, though, will be water. This is why, we think, you need to make sure you're having carbohydrates in the diet and a good amount of that too. Go to hodgsonhealth.com/macros to get it calculated for you (don't worry we won't put this link in again)

Once you have your calorie and macro goals, you're good to go, get them in the tracker (we suggest MyFitnessPal) and start eating your 'normal food', and track them accurately, then see how far away from your goals you are. Then adapt your food based on that.

Without going into too much depth because after all this isn't a science book. This is to help you understand the importance of nutrition in becoming the best you.

There are a couple of things you want to know about each of the macronutrients.

CARBOHYDRATES

Carbohydrates often get a bad run in the press. People often think that they are the enemy, always demonising them. They are the ones responsible for people being overweight. We have people tell us they only need to look at carbs and they gain weight.

However, this is really not the case. The reason people are overweight is that they're consuming more calories than they're burning. It's not one food, it's them all combined. When we look at carbohydrates, it's important to know that they are the body's primary source of energy. By energy, it's not just energy like if you're going out and doing exercise. It's energy as in for all the functions of the body. Your body's digestion is controlled by energy; your hormone production is controlled by energy, so you need to have a good supply of energy to be **the best version of yourself.** You cannot be the best colleague, the best parent, the best partner if you've not got the energy.

Your brain is controlled by energy. That energy comes from carbohydrates. In every gram of carbohydrate, there are four calories. Therefore, if you have 100 grams of carbohydrates in a day, there are 400 calories from the carbs alone.

It's important to know that generally speaking, a carbohydrate is a carbohydrate If you get 20 grams of carbohydrates from fruits such as a banana which will be mostly sugar-based carbohydrates, or you get 20 grams of carbohydrates from pasta, it's still the same number of calories, and this is all really what we need to remember when we're looking at our calories and macros.

You should not be cutting carbohydrates out of your diet. Yes, it's often said to avoid having peaks and troughs in your energy levels, having relatively small portions of carbohydrates can just help benefit that, however, there are also links to having fasting periods which help your body stabilise its blood sugar levels.

Carbohydrates play a massive role in the whole functioning of the body. Now we do know that some people can find they fluctuate in weight around carbohydrate consumption and linking it to insulin sensitivity, however when part of a balanced diet, it's rare that this is the case.

So again, you can argue either way. We need to keep things simple and just look at calories and getting the ratios right for you, and only you, which we will go onto after.

PROTEIN

Protein, again, is an extremely important nutrient. In fact, we're big fans of having a high protein diet for pretty much everyone, but particularly when trying to lose weight. Our rationale for this is simple.

Protein forms the building blocks behind the cells in the body, so as you can see, it is really important. From a weight-loss perspective it's also helpful as it takes longer for your body to metabolise, which has two profound benefits. The first one being, you'll feel a little fuller for longer. The second one being, if you consume them with carbohydrates, your body will take slightly longer to absorb those carbohydrates into the bloodstream, giving you more sustained energy.

This will mean that your energy levels will stay a little more consistent and you won't feel you crave that sugar fix, which can send many people toward making poor decisions.

The cells of the body have a protein molecule in them. So, as you can imagine, it's really important to make sure you have enough protein in your diet. There are four calories per gram of protein, exactly the same as carbohydrates.

Now, we've worked for several years with thousands of clients and some of them even being vegan and they still manage to get their protein levels up.

You can find protein in various plants based sources, too. It means you might need to eat a slightly higher volume of the food to get that protein up high enough. We find a western diet tends to be lower in Protein and higher in Fats and Carbs than we suggest for overall health.

Now, we always suggest a high protein diet and when we first do this with 9 out of the 10 men and women we speak to and explain to them the reasons a high protein diet is important, they often come back with the thought of a big gym type goer, and they will put loads of muscle on.

However, this is not the case. Most people, particularly, women aren't genetically geared to build muscle in that way. Protein is protein, it is not muscle. You are building those muscles based on hormones in the body with that protein. In fact, many of the women we work with end up having protein supplements to help get their protein up as part of their diet, they don't turn into bodybuilders overnight.

FATS

The last macronutrients are fats, another one of the macro nutrients that often gets a bad run of things. However, fats are absolutely vital for safe, long-term health.

Fats are vital and play a big part in the body. We need fats as a secondary energy source, exercises at a lower intensity will burn fat as an energy source as it takes longer to convert to energy in the body. They also absorb certain nutrients into the body, help protect your organs and even help maintain your body's temperature.

Now there are nine calories per gram of fat so you can imagine how quickly the calories will rack up on a high-fat diet. So we need the volume of fats to be kept low.

A good thing to keep in mind about Fats is you have a 'full switch' when you consume fats, whereas often we don't for carbohydrates.

The way we like to look at it is if you look at drinking a litre of fruit juice (which is mainly carbs), it's easy to drink. Your body can probably drink that without feeling too full. However, trying to drink a litre of full-fat milk, is a completely different feeling you'll experience, your body has a full switch for fats. So having fats in the diet can also be a good way to make sure you don't overeat.

Common Nutrition Mistakes

Some of the common mistakes we see when people are focusing on their diet include we see them eating a lot of foods which they deem 'healthy' and they are not in the right portion sizes.

However, as with everything we've discussed in this book, it's being aware of the nutritional values within the food you're eating.

We see this with foods like fruits, dried fruits avocados, peanut butter, and olive oils. People are doing it to think they're being healthy and consuming these types of foods.

However, they are actually a quick way for the calories to rack up through mindless eating or the mentality of 'oh it's healthy'. That's why eat what you like but track it, become aware of it and most of all make decisions around it based on your level of enjoyment, goals and lifestyle. It's just something to know of and think about when you look at your nutrients side of things. That's why we put such a strong emphasis on tracking your food so you can become more aware of what is in foods.

Now we sometimes get objections from people regarding tracking their food, which we totally get, but we are going to be very upfront here, if you don't want to track it's a strong indication you need to track even more so. You just know it will be uncomfortable to see how much you're consuming. Remember, don't judge yourself, it's a tool to help you.

Now there is a group of people who can perhaps have an obsessive relationship with tracking and if it ever feels unhealthy, we wouldn't advise tracking although we have had eating disorder survivors work with us on their mindset (albeit after they'd had treatment for their eating disorder) and get on very well with our tracking as its help to ensure they're eating enough too.

Now the reason we're so big on tracking your food is only to increase your understanding of what you're eating. Because we know knowledge and understanding are fundamental towards behaviour change.

That's what we're trying to do, is change your behaviour. Improve your eating habits, and adapt your eating patterns to become more aware of exactly what you're eating.

Once you become more aware of what you're eating, you'll make more conscious, healthier decisions. That's all we want from this part of the book, so if you get this, you're well on the way already.

ALCOHOL

Alcohol is something that always pops up when people are trying to lose weight because I think we all know deep down its empty calories. Per gram of alcohol there are 7 calories, so the calories will rack up quite quickly if you drink a lot of alcohol, and let's face it, you don't need a personal trainer or a coach, or a nutritional expert to tell you that alcohol isn't optimal to helping you from a holistic health perspective.

It can affect all 4 of the Bs when it comes to your goals, your body in the ways it makes keeping calories in check tougher, your brain as it can affect sleep, moods and generally how you feel, business from a lower energy perspective and besties from both moods and even a fulfillment perspective. Now we know that's not really helpful because, well many of us (yes us included) like a drink or two, and we also know a good night doesn't start with diet coke or sparkling water, it starts with bubbles and the alcoholic type for many occasions. So we don't want to encourage avoiding alcohol., especially if you do enjoy it.

We would, however, say awareness is key (yes again) for example, become aware of how many calories you're getting from alcohol. Say you drink five nights a week for example, and you reduce it down to two, you've made progress. You will make changes and feel the benefits from your sleep, moods, energy levels and much more, and that's more sustainable. That's why, we suggest that if you drink more then you should, reduce it, but you don't need to cut it out.

Because, again, like anything to do with diet, cutting it out is never going to be a good thing. All about balance and moderation. Sometimes switching drinks for lower calorie alcoholic drinks will be more beneficial for you, too, which you will establish when you start tracking because you're going to track, right?

However, we understand that alcohol is something that's not just a drink, it's the social ties that are attached to it and we don't believe that having goals should mean sacrificing enjoyment, if anything, they should add to it and a few drinks here and there will not negatively affect you.

THE SPLIT

Now by the split, we refer to is the ratio of Protein Carbs and Fats which we break down with clients after the calories are right. Now as previously mentioned, the carbs and fat ratio is less important than the protein one so let's work on that first. With the protein we tend to focus on increasing it as a start with aiming for 1.5 - 2g of protein to lbs of body weight. Whilst focusing on that protein content we would also try to keep the fats down a bit to leave more 'room' (calories) for carbohydrates.

Now we should say quickly, some people do respond better to higher fats and lower carbs, however from our experience this is the monitorty, and actually people tend to enjoy having more carbs in their diet both from a physical aspect in terms of energy, but also from an aspect of the enjoyment of their eating. So it's really important to take your time to track asses and adapt things to find out what suits you better.

When assessing it, don't just focus on the physical aspects such as energy, perhaps weight and shape, but also look at your moods, concentration 'get up and go' and generally how you feel as a whole.

Keep it simple, keep aware of it, and you can make your own decisions. You don't need a nutrition expert, or you don't need a coach such as us to tell you what to eat you know the answers.

Yes, you may need the right accountability and support when you're tracking it because you'll know straight away. In fact, we've lost count of the number of our clients that would message us after they've had a bad day, telling us what they did wrong. That's because they know they have the answers, it doesn't take a nutrition expert once you're tracking it because you'll become so much more aware.

That's why we say that knowledge is a huge part of the basics we all need. That is now made so much easier as we have tools like MyFitnessPal in place to make it almost foolproof.

ACTIVITY

SO NOW we've come to the activity part of this book, and in the past, we used to call this exercise, however now we know that exercise can often be an obstacle for people who are living a busy life. Although we would love everyone to be up for 'exercising' every day, we know it's not possible so we prefer to focus on the activity as a whole. We left this to last because once you have the mindset and lifestyle in place, let's face it the activity will be part of it because you'll have addressed the lifestyle which involves being active because you know being active will help-

- Reduced weight gain
- Increase moods
- Improve productivity
- Benefit sleep
- Reduced risk of heart disease

So we don't overly need to separate activity from lifestyle. However, it's the part that most people tend to focus on right from the start.

The first thing that people think of when they want to become the best version of themselves, particularly physically, is that they need to do more exercise, which nine times out of ten could be true, however like we've mentioned in every part of this book so far, it doesn't need to be extreme or complex.

In fact, far from it.

It doesn't need to be a complicated exercise plan that involves you spending hours and hours in the gym and missing out on your life that still carries on around you even when you're busy working towards your health and happiness goals.

We could probably end the activity part of the book right here because we know you've incorporated it as part of your lifestyle, right? But we will go over a few things to help you more specifically. But please don't over complicate things with this part as simplicity is easier to stick to.

Take small steps and move forward in just being more active. Whether that means as simple as parking the car further away from your work so you have to walk a little further, using the stairs instead of the lift, or walking to and from work. Even going to Zumba, if that's your thing, anything that burns more calories than sitting on your backside is a positive thing. We look at society now and can see it promotes us sitting down and getting things conveniently delivered to our doorstep.

We suggest hitting an average of 10k steps a day as a good guide to being active. One thing we see is a lot of people who train perhaps 4-5 days a week and call themselves active, yet spend 8-10 hours of their day behind a desk hardly moving so it's important to get a bit of perspective when it comes to activity levels. As training is just, say a maximum of an hour a day (this is longer than we ever train or have our clients train) the other 23 hours of the day are also part of determining whether you're active or not.

Now we would be lying if we tried to pretend that we didn't love the gym and wish that everyone could attend the gym to help them, but we know for many it's not realistic based on any of a number of things such as their schedule, confidence levels or commitments. However, if you can get to the gym or do some activity that involves weights, then you will definitely gain further benefits. However, you don't need to be going to a gym and beasting yourself for an hour at a time and walk out feeling like you're absolutely drained. When we did personal training face to face and even in our bootcamp and app now, we focus on giving a good intense workout targeting specific muscle groups so clients leave feeling worked out, but they have lives to get on with, so feeling like death is never the goal.

We really want to promote weights or resistance-based training regardless of your overall health goals. Lifting weights is going to help reduce muscle loss, improve hormone regulation, improve body shape and so much more. So even if your goal is to just run further and fast, still lift weights, we have clients running marathons and doing triathlons, lifting weights 3-5 times a week. It's important for injury prevention too and the bonus they've seen their times comes down too.

That's why we became more lifestyle based coaches over everything else because we found that it wasn't actually about the training sessions that people were struggling with. It was the other 23 or 23 and a half hours of the day. That's something we really want you to think about it, when you're training, yes, it's probably great. But that will not achieve anything unless the other 23+ hours of the day are good too.

That's why we focus so much on lifestyle. That's why we focused on mindset and that's why we focused on nutrition before we even mention activity or exercise. That's what we would need to remember when you go to focus on the activity or exercise in your life.

With being active it's important to think of heart health too because it's important to get the heart rate up regularly from, many of our clients have found by being more active they've been more productive with work, slept better, improved sex life, and are more fun to be around in general.

EXERCISE AND WEIGHT LOSS

We have to address weight loss and exercise because, well, in most of the western world, you're now part of the majority if you are overweight or obese, so we would hazard a guess that reading this, you'd like to lose a few lbs. Even if you wouldn't, this could still help.

When talking about exercise, we can easily categorise training into two key areas, resistance training, and cardiovascular training.

Resistance training is effectively putting some form of resistance against your muscles, which can either be as weights or bodyweight. Cardio training is effectively working your heart and lungs.

Now, the majority of people, when setting off on their weight loss journey will focus predominantly on cardio training because they perhaps thought it helps make them sweat more and they will burn more calories. Or because 'it worked last time'.

However, there is a lot of science behind the reasons resistance training being more beneficial, which is linked to what we discussed earlier about why everyone should do some form of resistance training and we'll get on to it more later in this chapter. Exercising and weight loss, we would say at first make sure you are increasing your level of activity as a whole.

In fact, with most of our coaching clients we just get them tracking their steps. It's as simple as that, which we covered in the lifestyle area, anyway.

But remember the absolute, most important part of exercise and increased body confidence is that you enjoy it.

Your life is for you so your goals should be for you too.

If you don't enjoy doing the form of exercise that you are doing now, or you've tried in the past, just don't do it- simple because it will only set you up to slip off the wagon at the first opportunity.

We also want to remove the relationship of using exercise as some form of punishment, we don't want you to turn to exercise just because you've had a big meal and feel like now you need to go for a run to burn it off. Everything you do in your lifestyle should be for enjoyment and feeling good. Remember, like we have said earlier one bad meal will not affect your progress just like one healthy meal won't either, we need to look long term, this is your lifestyle.

Yes, there are forms of exercise that will be better for helping you lose weight quicker. However, if you don't enjoy them, I can assure you they won't give you the long-term success you're looking for. We have lost count of the number of clients who have taken up running in the past to lose weight, picking up injuries and thinking they have to push on because 'running is the best way but it's really not. In fact if you struggle with body composition I'd guess you don't enjoy running, and running is only going to put further strain on your joints that are already carrying around extra weight.

So really, running is far from ideal, in fact, running would be way down the list of 'weight loss tools' with TeamHodgson

Be more patient and do something you enjoy. If you enjoy a particular form of exercise, then do it. If you enjoy circuit training, do circuit training. If you enjoy weight training, do weight training. If you enjoy swimming, go swimming. If you enjoy running, we guess we should say do running, but focus on form and some weights to build strength and reduce the risk of injury.

The key to it , really is enjoyment because then you won't resent your new found lifestyle and exercise within that.

If you spend time working towards your goals, doing things you don't enjoy, you are setting yourself up with an even longer battle with the scales .

So, try new things, try to think of it like this. The worst thing you will lose is a few weeks trying it. If you don't enjoy it, just change it, try something new. The beauty of the fitness industry now is that there are so many different ways to be active.

RESISTANCE TRAINING

When we speak about resistance training, often described as weights, many women will often think about a body builder or some big butch bloke or a big butch woman and think, *I don't want to get bulky.* (Yep, even Elly has done that in the past too)

However, there is a reason most women cannot get bulky. It's to do with women's hormones. Women aren't genetically designed to build muscle in the same way that a man would and even if they were, it would possibly benefit them with being lower in body fat, but many aren't. When you attain a body shape through lifting weights, you'll retain muscle and that muscle will burn calories. This is why we cannot stress enough to you how beneficial resistance-based training is compared to cardio-based. So, when we look at our resistance-based training, we want to be working the muscles to increase strength and if we can retain or even gain a bit of muscle, that would be of huge benefit to you, no doubt.

The reason we want to retain or put on muscle is one pound of muscle burns about 3,500 calories per week therefore, the more muscle we put on, the more calories we burn which means we can either eat more food, or find getting into a deficit easier. If you can increase your muscle mass, that will over time help you reduce your body fat.

You'll get to a point where your body won't continue to put on muscle, but that muscle will still be there burning calories. Another thing to remember is that muscle is more dense than fat.

So by this, we mean one pound of muscle will take up a lot less room than a pound of fat, which means shape change. As we know from experience that often when we talk to people about weight loss, it's not just about the number on the scales, it's about appearance. So, get those before pictures, track your confidence levels, assess how you feel then adapt based on that. Yet we did it again, **Track, Assess, Adapt**, that is your gauge.

So, when we talk about resistance training or weights, it's important to remember that we really want to try to target the bigger muscle groups.

So by this, we mean hitting your legs, your glutes (bum), chest, shoulders and back. These are the muscles that will burn more calories and usually will be enough to see great physical progress and psychological benefits too.

Doing loads of abdominal work and crunches will burn minimal calories, and you cannot spot reduce.

Spot reducing is where if you work a muscle group, you will burn fat on top of it. However, this is not the case. Muscle doesn't choose where it burns fat from, it burns calories, and the calories we utilise — the body will utilise the calories from wherever it sees fit.

In fact, more often than not, the first place you want to lose the body fat/weight from is the last place it comes off, frustrating, but true. So you need to have a little bit of patience (yes, patience again). The shape will change over time and the results will be long lasting.

So when you're looking at resistance training, it's important to remember that muscles will pull. They pull to contract, to create movement at a joint (for example, the bicep pulls to close the joint at the elbow) as in lift weights, but they will also pull you around in posture.

Therefore, it's important to get a balanced program when you do weights. You're working the front muscles just as much as you work the back muscles unless you have a postural problem, then you might need to have a stronger focus on certain muscle groups. But this is really important, particularly for long term health. With many in sitting jobs or on their computers and laptops phones etc, it's quite common now to see people with drawn forward shoulders which is not ideal from a body shape perspective, but also from an energy perspective, or lower back issues which can arise from rounded shoulders.

Once you've established that, we always recommend splitting the body into different muscle groups or body parts so that then you're resting some on other days and working others throughout the body. But again, this depends on how often you can fit having weights into your lifestyle.

For rep range, (by rep range we mean the amount of times you lift the weights before putting them down). We always suggest getting enough reps to keep the weights under tension for at least 30 seconds but possibly longer, so a lot of the work we do is 12-20 reps. By the end of the desired reps it should be a struggle. If it was easy, we normally suggest going heavier but not too heavy to sacrifice form and technique. Keep the rest nice and short and that will keep the heart rate nice and high, too. Once we do that, you're actually going to work your cardiovascular system anyway which we'll cover briefly further on.

When you do weights, it's important to remember that technique is everything, doing it safely, and starting off light, building the weight up as you get more confident and the weights become easier, as a beginner even starting with the machines to get the confidence up, it will benefit you in the long term.

If you're unsure on how to lift the weights correctly, get help from somebody (or try our app for FREE at hodgsonhealth.com/trial) who knows what they're doing because it's so easy to injure yourself by lifting weights with improper form.

When trying to lose weight, doing body weight workouts or circuits can be just as effective as lifting heavy weights, especially if you are lower in confidence, extremely busy or just don't feel like going to the gym.

You should never feel pressured into going to a gym, particularly if it will make you feel unhappy, stressed and affect the quality of your workout. However, we will say from our experience training in many gyms people are generally very supportive in them and as the old saying goes 'we all start somewhere'.

We also know what stress does to results now- (if not, refer back to mindset and lifestyle).

We know it's not practical for everyone to get into a gym, for many different reasons,in fact, when a majority of our clients actually do their workouts from home. We suggest doing it in a circuit format where you have perhaps a set time frame for exercises or much higher reps to get the intensity up.

Generally, we suggest splitting the body up over days to ensure you hit all the bigger muscle groups however if time is limited and you have a day or two between workouts, you could do whole body workouts. Particularly as a beginner. I think at first, looking at what is going to help you best and doing full body workouts can mean you perhaps don't quite ache as much so it doesn't affect the rest of your life. With the ache, it's called DOMS delayed onset muscle soreness some people get it all the time while some don't. It's not an indicator of working hard, it's just how we recover. Plenty of water, keep moving and adequate protein in your diet and the DOMS will subside before too long.

Again, there should always be a strong focus on form and technique to make sure you will not injure yourself, and if you're unsure, always ask for help.

There's so much information out there now that you can go online and find out how to perform exercises in a safe and controlled manner.

We suggest you spend a little bit of time educating yourself on doing that, so you don't pick up injuries. Or you can of course get our app for that help too.

CARDIO

SO, WHEN YOU first set out on your pursuit of self-progress, and you're working on the exercise side of things, it's easy to fall into the trap of doing more and more cardio. Which is great provided it fits your lifestyle and you enjoy it.

So, going out and doing the cardio is fine. However, there are a few things to remember when doing loads of cardio. One of the main things to remember is that your appetite can and will increase. In fact, there are various studies out there that prove that people who do more cardio, tend to eat more, so become aware that when doing more cardio you may start to feel more hungry, and this is ok because you're burning more but you don't want this to have a negative impact on your goals.

So, there's no point in doing a cardio workout, burning an extra 400 calories, and then eating an extra 500 calories without thinking about it or 'because you need it' or even worse to reward yourself, unless of course, you want to gain weight,because you've just almost wasted that workout particularly if the cardio was a low intensity 'calorie' burn like most people do 'cardio.'

That's why we put such a strong emphasis on doing resistance training, something to consider is that when you work on cardio, if you're somebody who's overweight, remember things like jogging and running and even brisk walking can put a lot of stress and impact on the joints, in particular, the lower back, hips, and knees.

So, you need to bear that in mind, if you want to do the cardio, to build it up slowly. Don't go from doing nothing to hammering the cardio every day because your joints will be absolutely shot.

We need to ease yourself into the impact, so that over time, they become used to it. And also, as the weight comes off you (which if you have the mindset, lifestyle and nutrition right, it will), there will be less impact travelling through your joints.

Now, often when people talk about cardio training, they think it's just going out running or walking on a treadmill, on a bike, something that's relatively low in intensity and just continuous, which is fine to do if you have a goal that is relevant to running for a long time or an endurance-based event.

However, the term cardio comes from the word cardiovascular, which is your heart and lungs. Therefore, when we are doing any form of cardio training, we should aim to get the heart and lungs working nice and hard.

That's right, your heart is a muscle, so we want to make sure we're working that muscle to improve its strength and performance, which of course, will come with a whole host of benefits. Now, when we say that, there are different ways to do this. There is, steady state where you get your heart rate to a moderate intensity and keep it there. Then there's interval training, where we work at a higher intensity for a period, lower intensity or rest period.

For us, we find that time is often an issue, therefore doing high-intensity interval training, also known as HIIT, is the best form to keep time to a minimum. You can do an intensive HIIT training session and it can be over within about 10 to 12 minutes, providing you're going high intensity to your fitness levels.

HIIT is a type of interval training where we go to a high intensity with minimal rest before getting the intensity up again.

Remember, anything should be done by your fitness levels and your fitness levels only. SO if you do go down the HIIT workouts like we have on our app, it is important to listen to your body and work yourself up. You can be the fittest guy going and struggle in a HIIT 12 minutes workout .This is what cardio training is.

Now, if you will do the long, slow stuff, it's only effective if you're doing it as burning extra calories or simply for enjoyment which is absolutely fine.

Especially if you have a weight loss goal, but that's where we would always suggest just be more active in life (refer back to lifestyle). It could be to go out for a walk with the kids or with the dog. It could be out running, playing football with the kids. It could even just be using stairs instead of the lift. Parking the car slightly further away in the car parks, so you have a little more distance to travel. You get our drift by now, right? you haven't read this far and not got that?.

So, Enjoy being active and if you're doing cardio....

KEEP IT INTENSE FOR YOU

As we've already mentioned with the weights side of things, you can get a good cardio workout by doing resistance based training and keep your weights heavy (for you) and your recovery short. Now you know all cardio is just keeping a heart rate nice and high.

You're wondering now you're coming towards the end of this book what do you have to do now?

We thought we could make an exhaustive list to make it really simple.

First things first, you need to go out and get yourself a good notepad you really value. Remember, the more expensive it is, the more you invest in it, the more you will respect it and use it. We heard the saying before: **the more you pay, the more you pay attention.**

Then you need to set some goals out. Remember, you need to do the homework as to why those goals are important. Use your notepad and pen, write out your goals and why they're important.

- **Remember, goals have a deadline.**

At the beginning of this book, we promised you we'd give you an easy-to-follow formula that would ultimately give you sustainable lifelong progress.

But not just any old sustainable progress, sustainable progress in a way that means you don't feel you're impacting your life in a negative way, you want to add value to it.

One that works by having and understanding the importance of having balance in your life. The last thing we want to do is add chaos to it.

So, do these simple things every single day, and we guarantee you will see great progress. It's not just physical progress; **it will be mental progress, too.**

1. Daily rituals: Yes, they are important. In fact, they are vital. They will help you become and remain aligned with your goals every single day. We're reminding you how important they are and to keep working towards them, no matter what life throws at you. And even when you think you have it all under control, don't let these slip. We often chat to people who suddenly find they've lost their clarity or motivation, then we ask if they're still journaling, and they'd let it slip.

2. Daily gratitude: Yes, every single day, we want you to think about what you're grateful for in the world, no matter how big or how small, hold on to that gratitude and feel it. When was the last time you sat down and literally appreciated the positive things that are going on in your life? No matter how big or how small, do this daily. It will make you appreciate things so much more because there are always things we can be positive and grateful for, when we learn to find them and connect with them emotionally. Not just sitting there saying 'i'm grateful', FEEL IT!

3. Activity: Be active at some point every single day. Most of our clients have done the 10 to 12-minute workouts during the day. It's easy to fit in from a lifestyle point of view, and they're doing something every single day in a positive way to help towards their goals. This will become a habit quite quickly. But if that's not for you, just think 'I want to get my heart rate up for at least a few minutes today'.

4. Journaling Or tracking: We want you to journal everything, from what you're eating to how you're feeling to what progress you've made. Why? Because we know if you're not tracking it's difficult to make smaller changes with confidence. You may have heard the saying if you're not assessing, you're guessing and we want to take the guesswork out of it so you have a clear path. You have a clear way you've progressed and a way you haven't, so you know things that need to work on.

5. Nutrition: We want you to have it in mind of what you're eating, become more aware of it, track it if you can, then you can assess and adapt as you see fit. We don't want you to ever feel you're on a diet but we want you to know that you can use nutrition to help you FEEL BETTER. Think performance for life, with goals in them 4Bs you want to have energy and nourishing your body is key to this.

6. Lifestyle: We want you to attempt to become slightly more active in your lifestyle every single day. This might just be as simple as using stairs instead of the lift, parking slightly further away from work. The more active you are the better you will feel and the more calories you will burn which will help maintain a body you want whilst consuming more food.

7. Personal development: Personal development is a key part of you, improving yourself as a person, physically and mentally. We know like we've said at several points throughout this book, the mind will always lead the body, so get the mind working and get yourself developed in a mental way so that your body can then start developing itself too. Condition the brain first, the mind leads the body. It could be 3-5 minutes a day of videos to help or reading a book to learn and APPLY IT.

Bonus side note: Plan the time in your day from waking up to going to sleep. This will help you find spare time for you to commit to doing things that will help you become the best version of yourself. Look at your lifestyle and see if there are things you're perhaps wasting time with that you can remove from your day and take control of the direction you're heading.

Remember, if it doesn't serve you and it's not a necessity, you can remove it from your day, having no major impacts on yourself and don't feel guilty about that.

You now have all the tools to move forward with your goals. We can make it into a game like we do with our clients.

THE BEST VERSION OF YOURSELF GAME

THAT IS RIGHT: we want it to become a game and make it a little more fun, how many times has it become a chore in the past trying to work towards that goal, to get that next promotion, that improved relationship, lose that weight.

We find one sure-fire way to make sure you stay making progress when looking towards your weight loss goals is to 'Gamify' it. Create a sort of game with a points system that works for you.

For us, we have points in all four areas we covered in this book (sure you will do too now). We have points for mindset, lifestyle, nutrition and activity. The reason we do this is it motivates us to make sure we do something each day that focuses us to gain points.

We give ourselves a target to get once we get a set amount of points. It could be a date night or some new clothing.

What you'll find, once you start to do that, you can really keep motivated, and it also can become a fun thing within the family.

We count points every week and journal it (yes, that shiny journal you bought at the start of this book, wink wink). Give this a go and you'll see how much more motivated you are.

You only have to look at various other things that work on points, such as Weight Watchers and how successful it is, because people love counting points. We all love making games out of things and we want to win. So, let's try to win at being our best, win at our lifestyle, and win at this game.

Remember, points make prizes and the best prize of all-the incredible self-progress that will come with it and seems effortless too.

We have a 5-points system in our group which we regularly work with on our clients; we play 35 points for the week.

1- Daily rituals and gratitude and even personal development.

2- 30 minutes activity every day (just the heart rate raised)

3- Taking photos of food and putting it in our group (you can do it publicly. This will help you choose wisely)

4- Being within your calorie goal.

5- We have an activity, exercise or challenge of the week to keep it active.

So this is something we do with our clients and we have noticed a huge positive change in their commitment and motivation. It also makes things fun as often enough, the reason we stop doing certain things is that we do not enjoy it. So set yourself a target for the first week of how many points you will aim for? Perhaps do it with your peer group (or with TeamHodgson)

We hope you have gained from this book and can see the importance of working on the 4 key principles but also setting yourself goals within the 4Bs of life.

A HUGE THANK YOU

WE WANT TO sign this book off by saying a huge thank you.

Thanking you for investing your time, your money and your energy into reading this book. We know you have a busy life, and there are thousands of books you could have read, but you chose ours.

We hope that you have taken something valuable away from it whether it be regarding mindset, lifestyle, nutrition or activity.

We hope you'll walk away from reading this book feeling like you've learned something and feel one step closer to becoming the best version of you.

We hope this book will be something that is going to not only help you short-term but help you longer term and even those around you too.

Because we know when you are in a better place, everyone else around you benefits. As a thank you all, we will offer you a free 30-minute coaching call worth £199. All you have to do is give us a 5-star rating on Amazon and tag us on your stories @RyanHodgsonFitness @EllyHodgsonFitness

We really value every single person who takes the time to read this book, and will personally read EVERY review. If you learnt something from it, send us a note. Include exactly what you learnt, so we can help more people on their journey.

We're always keen to connect with readers of the book and hear their progress. So, please let us know how you find it, what progress you make, and we look forward to hearing from you.

Once you finish with this book, gift it to somebody. Spread the knowledge and spread the passion we have for helping women become the best version of themselves.

So thank you once again for taking the time out of your busy schedule to read this book. We are eternally grateful to you and hope that the lesson you've learned from it will continue to help you for the rest of your life.

Ryan and Elly xx

ABOUT RYAN & ELLY

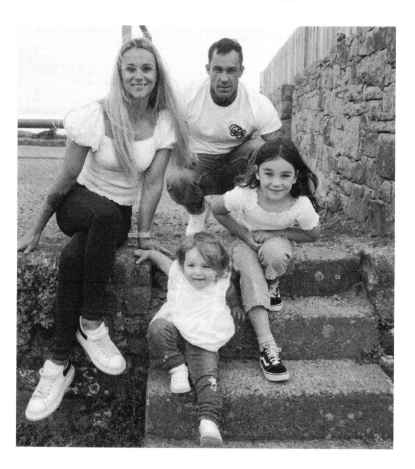

Ryan and Elly Hodgson are online coaches, bootcamp owners living in Jersey with their two girls Aoife-Mae (6) and Niamh (2) and dog Alfie. They've been married for 5 years and have a combined knowledge of over 15 years in the industry.

Elly has a Sport Science with Psychology degree and is pre and post natal qualified. Ryan has level 3 Psychology Human Biology and furthered his nutrition specialist. They've worked online for the last 5 years and have helped over 2500 people toward their goals.

CONNECT WITH US

A few links may be of interest. We would love to connect with you:

Our Instagram and Facebook pages—we always want to connect with people

Instagram.com/RyanHodgsonFitness

Instagram.,com/EllyHodgsonFitness

Facebook.com/RyanHodgsonFitness

Facebook.com/EllyHodgsonFitness

Facebook.com/RyanAndElly

Our website

You can go to Hodgsonhealth.com/trial to join our programme and get a 7 day free trial. Then be in TeamHodgson for under £2 a day.

Or email either us at

Ryan@HodgsonFitness.com

Elly@HodgsonFitness.com

We look forward to connecting with you.

Printed in Great Britain
by Amazon

55446236R00084